Fitness for Seniors: How 5 Minutes Can Restore Your Balance, Energy, and Sense of Humor

By

Jordan Rivers

Copyright 2024

All rights reserved.

ISBN: 9798877227682
Imprint: Independently published

<u>DEDICATION</u>

To all seniors who, like me, need motivation, guidance, exercise, and a better sense of humor about aging!

CONTENTS

Introduction

As we age, our bodies undergo various changes, and staying fit and healthy becomes increasingly important. Exercise plays a vital role in maintaining physical and mental well-being, yet many seniors find it challenging to incorporate fitness into their daily lives. If you're a senior looking for a simple and effective way to improve your balance, energy levels, and overall sense of humor, you've come to the right place.

Welcome to "Easy Fitness for Seniors: How 5 Minutes Can Restore Your Balance, Energy, and Sense of Humor."

In this book, we will explore the power of short and efficient workouts that require only five minutes of your day. Yes, you read it correctly—just five minutes! This book is designed to prove that it's never too late to start exercising and that even the shortest bursts of physical activity can have significant benefits.

In the following chapters, we will delve into the world of senior fitness, both from the seniors' point-of-view as well as the people who are looking to help them, all the while learning the unique challenges seniors face and the countless advantages of exercise for their well-being. We will introduce you to the concept of a 5-minute fitness routine, which is not only manageable but also incredibly effective for seniors of all fitness levels.

Throughout this book, you'll discover that achieving optimal health doesn't have to be a time-consuming or complex endeavor. We will guide you through the essential components of a 5-minute fitness routine, which include warm-up exercises, low-impact cardiovascular activities, strength training movements, flexibility exercises, and stress-relieving cool-downs. You will learn how to tailor your routine to suit your abilities and individual needs, ensuring a safe yet invigorating workout experience.

We also understand the importance of having fun while exercising, especially when it comes to seniors. Laughter is a powerful tool that promotes overall wellness, and we will explore how to incorporate joy and humor into your fitness routine. By finding delight in the process, you'll look forward to your workouts and reap even greater rewards for your mind, body, and soul.

Additionally, we will discuss strategies to stay motivated and consistent along your fitness journey. From setting realistic goals to creating a supportive environment, we will equip you with the tools needed to stay on track and celebrate each milestone you achieve.

Finally, we will provide additional tips and resources to help you maintain a healthy and active lifestyle outside of your 5-minute fitness routine. From overall wellness recommendations for seniors to exploring technology and fitness apps designed specifically for your needs, there is a wealth of knowledge waiting to support you.

So, are you ready to embark on a transformative journey that requires only five minutes of your time? Let's prove that age is just a number, and that easy fitness can truly restore your balance, energy, and sense of humor. Whether you're a fitness enthusiast or a beginner, this book will empower you to take control of your health and embrace a more vibrant and fulfilling senior lifestyle.

A. Importance of exercise for seniors

Exercise plays a crucial role in promoting optimal health and well-being for people of all ages, including seniors. In fact, maintaining an active lifestyle becomes even more important as we age. Regular exercise offers numerous benefits that can enhance the physical, mental, and emotional health of seniors, enabling them to lead fulfilling and independent lives.

1. Physical Health:

a. Improved Balance and Stability: Engaging in exercises that focus on balance and coordination can help prevent falls, a common concern among seniors. Strengthening core muscles and improving stability can significantly reduce the risk of injuries.

b. Increased Strength and Flexibility:
Regular physical activity helps build and maintain muscle strength, which is crucial for performing daily tasks and maintaining independence. Flexibility exercises can enhance mobility and range of motion, making activities like bending, reaching, and walking easier and more comfortable.

c. Enhanced Cardiovascular Health:
Cardio exercises, such as brisk walking or swimming, can improve heart and lung health, reducing the risk of heart disease, high blood pressure, and stroke. Increased cardiovascular fitness also leads to improved endurance and stamina in daily activities.

2. <u>Mental and Cognitive Health:</u>

a. Reduced Risk of Cognitive Decline:
Research suggests that exercise can help reduce the risk of cognitive decline and conditions like Alzheimer's disease. Regular physical activity promotes blood flow to the brain, stimulating the growth of new brain cells and improving cognitive function.

b. Boosted Mood and Emotional Well-being:
Exercise triggers the release of endorphins, also known as "feel-good" hormones, leading to improved mood and reduced symptoms of anxiety and depression. Seniors who engage in regular exercise often report greater happiness and improved overall emotional well-being.

c. Sharpened Mental Acuity:
Physical activity improves cognitive abilities such as memory, attention, and problem-solving skills. By stimulating the brain's neural connections, exercise can help seniors stay mentally sharp and maintain cognitive functioning.

3. Quality of Life:

a. Increased Independence: By improving strength, balance, and flexibility, seniors can enhance their ability to perform daily activities independently, reducing dependence on others and maintaining a higher quality of life.

b. Enhanced Energy and Vitality:
Regular exercise boosts energy levels and reduces fatigue, increasing overall vitality and stamina. This, in turn, allows seniors to engage in enjoyable activities, spend quality time with loved ones, and pursue their passions.

c. Social Engagement and Sense of Community:
Participating in group exercise classes or activities promotes social interaction, fostering a sense of community and combating feelings of loneliness or isolation.

Exercise is of utmost importance for seniors. By incorporating regular physical activity into their lives, seniors can experience improved balance, increased strength, and flexibility, enhanced cardiovascular health, better cognitive function, boosted mood and emotional well-being, increased independence, and an overall higher quality of life. Remember, it's never too late to start exercising, and even small amounts of activity can make a significant difference in seniors' well-being and longevity.

Benefits of incorporating a fitness routine into daily life

Incorporating a fitness routine into daily life offers a wide array of benefits for individuals of all ages. By committing to regular exercise, you can experience positive changes that contribute to a healthier, more fulfilling lifestyle. Here are some key benefits of incorporating a fitness routine into your daily life:

1. Improved Physical Health:

a. Weight Management: Regular exercise helps burn calories and build muscle, which can assist in maintaining a healthy weight and preventing obesity.

b. Stronger Muscles and Bones:

Strength training exercises promote muscle growth and enhance bone density, reducing the risk of conditions like osteoporosis and improving overall physical strength.

c. Enhanced Cardiovascular Health:

Engaging in cardiovascular exercises, such as jogging, swimming, or cycling, improves heart health, lowers blood pressure, and reduces the risk of cardiovascular diseases.

2. Increased Energy Levels:

Regular physical activity boosts energy levels by improving blood circulation, increasing oxygen and nutrient delivery to the muscles and organs, and enhancing overall stamina. With increased energy, you'll be better equipped to tackle daily tasks and enjoy recreational activities.

3. Mental Well-being:

a. Reduced Stress and Anxiety:
Exercise stimulates the production of endorphins, which are natural mood enhancers. Regular physical activity can lower stress levels, alleviate anxiety, and improve overall mental well-being.

b. Improved Cognitive Function:
Research suggests that exercise has positive effects on cognitive function, including memory, attention, and problem-solving abilities. Regular exercise can enhance brain health and may even help prevent cognitive decline.

c. Better Sleep:

Regular physical activity can promote better sleep quality, helping you fall asleep faster and enjoy deeper, more restorative sleep.

4. Disease Prevention and Management:

a. Chronic Disease Prevention:
Regular exercise plays a crucial role in preventing chronic conditions such as heart disease, type 2 diabetes, certain types of cancer, and metabolic disorders.

b. Management of Existing Conditions:
Exercise can enhance the management and control of chronic conditions, including arthritis, high blood pressure, and chronic pain, by reducing symptoms and improving overall functional abilities.

5. <u>Boosted Mood and Emotional Well-being:</u>

Engaging in physical activity releases endorphins, which are natural mood boosters. Regular exercise can reduce the risk of depression, alleviate symptoms of anxiety and stress, and promote a more positive outlook on life.

6. Enhanced Longevity:

Studies consistently indicate that individuals who incorporate regular exercise into their daily routines tend to live longer than those who lead sedentary lifestyles. Exercise contributes to overall health and vitality, reducing the risk of premature mortality.

7. <u>Social Engagement and Community:</u>

Participating in group exercises, fitness classes, or team sports creates opportunities for social interaction and fosters a sense of community. This can enhance feelings of belonging, combat loneliness, and provide a support network for individuals on their fitness journey.

Incorporating a fitness routine into your daily life isn't just about physical transformation; it's about embracing a healthier, more fulfilling lifestyle. By prioritizing regular exercise, you can experience improved physical health, increased energy levels, enhanced mental well-being, disease prevention and management, boosted mood, longevity, and opportunities for social engagement. Remember, consistency and finding activities you enjoy are key to making exercise a sustainable and enjoyable part of your daily life.

C. Overview of the 5-minute fitness concept

The 5-minute fitness concept is a revolutionary approach to exercise that focuses on short, intense workouts designed to be completed in just five minutes. This concept acknowledges the busy lives we lead and recognizes that finding time for exercise can be a challenge. However, it also emphasizes that even a brief burst of physical activity can yield significant benefits for our health and well-being.

The idea behind the 5-minute fitness concept is to provide a realistic and achievable exercise routine that can easily be incorporated into our daily lives. The aim is to eliminate the common excuse of not having enough time for exercise by demonstrating that just five minutes can make a positive impact on our fitness levels.

These short and efficient workouts are designed to maximize results by incorporating exercises that target various aspects of fitness, including cardiovascular endurance, strength, flexibility, and balance. Each workout is carefully curated and structured to ensure that every minute of those precious five minutes is utilized effectively.

The beauty of the 5-minute fitness concept lies in its versatility and adaptability. Whether you are a young adult, a busy professional, or a senior, the routines can be tailored to your specific needs and abilities. The exercises can be modified to accommodate different fitness levels, ensuring that everyone, regardless of their current condition, can benefit from this approach.

The 5-minute fitness concept aims at breaking down the misconception that exercise must be time-consuming or complicated. It encourages individuals to embrace the idea that every little bit of physical activity counts towards improved health. By integrating short bursts of exercise throughout the day, individuals can reap the rewards of increased energy levels, improved cardiovascular health, enhanced strength and mobility, and a boosted sense of well-being.

In the following chapters of this book, we will explore the essential components of a 5-minute fitness routine, provide guidance on tailoring the routine to individual needs, discuss how to infuse fun and humor into exercise and offer tips for staying motivated and consistent. Together, we will discover how dedicating just five minutes to fitness each day can lead to an overall transformation of our physical and mental well-being.

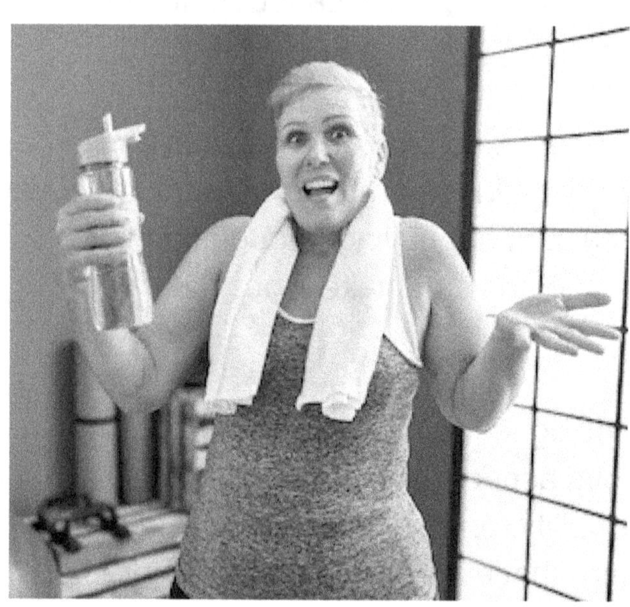

Chapter 1: Understanding Senior Fitness

As we age, our bodies undergo various changes, and it becomes increasingly important to prioritize our overall health and well-being. Regular exercise and physical activity play a crucial role in maintaining optimal fitness levels, functionality, and quality of life for seniors. Understanding senior fitness involves recognizing the unique challenges faced by older adults and implementing appropriate exercise strategies to address these concerns.

1. Common Challenges Faced by Seniors:

a. Decreased Muscle Mass:
Aging is associated with a natural decline in muscle mass, strength, and flexibility. This can lead to reduced mobility, increased risk of falls, and difficulty performing daily activities.

b. Decreased Bone Density:
Osteoporosis, a condition characterized by weak and brittle bones, becomes more prevalent with age, increasing the risk of fractures and injuries.

c. Declining Balance and Coordination:
Loss of balance and coordination make seniors more susceptible to falls, which can have severe consequences for their overall well-being.

d. Joint Pain and Stiffness:
Conditions such as arthritis can cause joint pain, stiffness, and reduced range of motion, making exercise challenging for seniors.

e. Chronic Health Conditions:
Many seniors experience chronic health conditions such as cardiovascular disease, diabetes, and high blood pressure, which may require considerations when designing a fitness routine.

2. Benefits of Exercise for Seniors:
a. Improved Functional Capacity:

Regular exercise helps maintain and improve strength, flexibility, and balance, enabling seniors to carry out daily activities with greater independence and ease.

b. Enhanced Bone Health:
Weight-bearing exercises and strength training can help maintain or increase bone density, reducing the risk of fractures and osteoporosis in seniors.

c. Increased Cardiovascular Fitness:
Engaging in aerobic exercises, such as walking, cycling, or swimming, improves heart health, circulation, and stamina, reducing the risk of cardiovascular diseases.

d. Mood and Cognitive Benefits:
Exercise stimulates the release of endorphins, promoting positive moods and reducing symptoms of depression and anxiety. Physical activity is also associated with improved cognitive function and a decreased risk of cognitive decline.

e. Chronic Disease Management:
Regular exercise can help manage chronic conditions such as arthritis, diabetes, and high blood pressure by improving symptoms, reducing medication reliance, and enhancing overall well-being.

3. <u>Safety Considerations for Exercising as a Senior:</u>

a. Consultation with Healthcare Professionals: Before starting any exercise program, it is essential for seniors to consult with their healthcare provider, especially if they have any underlying health conditions or concerns.

b. Proper Warm-up and Cool-down:
Seniors should incorporate a warm-up routine to prepare the body for exercise and a cool-down to gradually lower heart rate and prevent muscle soreness.

c. Balance and Stability Training:

Exercises to improve balance and stability should be included to reduce the risk of falls. These may involve standing on one leg, heel-to-toe walks, or specific balance training exercises.

d. Modified Exercises:
Seniors should choose exercises that are appropriate for their fitness level and modify them as needed to accommodate any joint pain or limitations.

e. Adequate Rest and Recovery:
Older adults may require longer recovery periods between workouts to avoid overexertion and allow the body to adapt and repair.

Understanding senior fitness involves acknowledging the unique challenges faced by older adults and developing exercise routines that address their specific needs. By engaging in regular exercise, seniors can experience improved functional capacity, enhanced bone health, increased cardiovascular fitness, positive mood and cognitive benefits, and better management of chronic conditions. With proper guidance and consideration of safety factors, seniors can maintain an active and healthy lifestyle well into their golden years.

A. <u>Common challenges faced by seniors</u>

Here are a few common challenges that seniors may encounter:

1. Physical Limitations:
Seniors may have limitations due to age-related health conditions, such as arthritis, osteoporosis, or chronic pain. These conditions can make certain exercises more challenging or uncomfortable.

2. Lack of Mobility:
Mobility issues can restrict the types of exercises seniors can perform. Conditions like joint stiffness or muscle weakness may make activities like walking, running, or lifting weights difficult.

3. Fear of Injury:

Seniors may have a fear of falling or getting injured while exercising. This fear can prevent them from engaging in physical activities or trying new exercises.

4. Lack of Knowledge:
Some seniors may be unaware of appropriate exercise techniques or the latest research on senior fitness. They may hesitate to start exercising due to a lack of knowledge about safe and effective practices.

5. Lack of Motivation:
Seniors may struggle with staying motivated to exercise regularly. This can be due to factors such as feeling tired, lack of social support, or a perceived lack of immediate benefits.

6. Financial Constraints:
Costly gym memberships or exercise equipment may pose a challenge for seniors on a limited budget. This can limit their access to exercise resources and facilities.

It's important to note that these challenges can vary among individuals, and it's always recommended to consult with a healthcare professional or a qualified fitness instructor who can provide guidance tailored to individual needs.

B. <u>Benefits of exercise for physical and mental health</u>

Exercise offers numerous benefits for both physical and mental health in seniors. Here are some key benefits:

1. Improved Cardiovascular Health:
Regular exercise can strengthen the heart, improve circulation, and lower the risk of cardiovascular diseases like heart disease and stroke.

2. Increased Strength and Flexibility:
Engaging in exercises that promote muscle strength and flexibility, such as resistance training and stretching, can help seniors maintain or improve their overall physical mobility and independence.

3. Better Bone Health:
Weight-bearing exercises, like walking or dancing, can help promote bone density and reduce the risk of osteoporosis and fractures.

4. Enhanced Balance and Fall Prevention:
Exercises that focus on balance, coordination, and stability, such as tai chi or yoga, can help reduce the risk of falls and improve overall balance.

5. Disease Prevention:
Regular physical activity can reduce the risk of chronic diseases like diabetes, certain types of cancer, and age-related conditions such as dementia.

<u>Mental Health Benefits</u>:

1. Stress Relief:
Exercise can help reduce stress levels and promote relaxation, contributing to an improved overall sense of well-being.

2. Improved Mood:
Physical activity stimulates the release of endorphins, which are natural mood boosters. Regular exercise can help reduce symptoms of anxiety and depression.

3. Enhanced Cognitive Function:
Exercise has been shown to have a positive impact on cognitive function and can help improve memory, attention, and overall brain health in seniors.

4. Social Engagement:
Participating in group exercise classes or activities can provide seniors with social interaction, reducing feelings of isolation and improving mental well-being.

5. Increased Self-Esteem and Confidence:
Regular exercise can improve self-esteem and promote positive body image, contributing to a greater sense of confidence in seniors.

It's important for seniors to consult with their healthcare provider before starting any new exercise program and to choose activities that suit their capabilities and preferences.

C. <u>Safety considerations for exercising as a senior</u>

When it comes to exercising as a senior, safety should always be a top priority. Here are some essential safety considerations to keep in mind:

1. Consult with a Healthcare Professional:
Before starting any new exercise program, it's crucial to consult with a healthcare provider or a qualified fitness professional. They can assess your overall health and provide guidance on exercises that are safe and suitable for you.

2. Start Slowly and Progress Gradually:
If you're new to exercise or have been inactive for a while, it's important to start with low-impact activities and gradually increase the intensity and duration. This allows your body to adapt and reduces the risk of injuries.

3. Warm-up and Cool Down:
Always begin your exercise routine with a proper warm-up session to prepare your muscles and joints for activity. Similarly, finish with a cool-down period to gradually bring your heart rate down and prevent dizziness or lightheadedness.

4. Use Proper Form and Technique:
Learning and using correct form and technique during exercises is essential for preventing injuries. If you're unsure about how to perform a specific exercise, consider seeking guidance from a qualified fitness professional.

5. Stay Hydrated:
Dehydration can occur more easily in seniors, so it's important to drink enough water before, during, and after exercise to maintain hydration.

6. Listen to your Body:
Pay attention to any discomfort, pain, or unusual symptoms during exercise. If you experience chest pain, severe shortness of breath, dizziness, or any other concerning symptoms, stop exercising and seek medical attention.

7. Wear Appropriate Clothing and Footwear:
Choose comfortable clothing that allows for ease of movement and proper footwear that provides stability and support. This can help prevent accidents and falls.

8. Consider Environmental Factors:
Be mindful of the exercise environment. Exercise in well-lit areas, avoid slippery or uneven surfaces and be cautious of extreme weather conditions to reduce the risk of accidents.

9. Modify or Avoid High-Risk Exercises:
Certain exercises may pose higher risks for seniors, especially those with pre-existing health conditions or physical limitations. Modify or avoid exercises that involve heavy weights, high-impact movements, or excessive joint stress if they are not suitable for your situation.

Remember, everyone's physical capabilities and health status are unique, so it's important to work with professionals who can provide personalized guidance and recommendations.

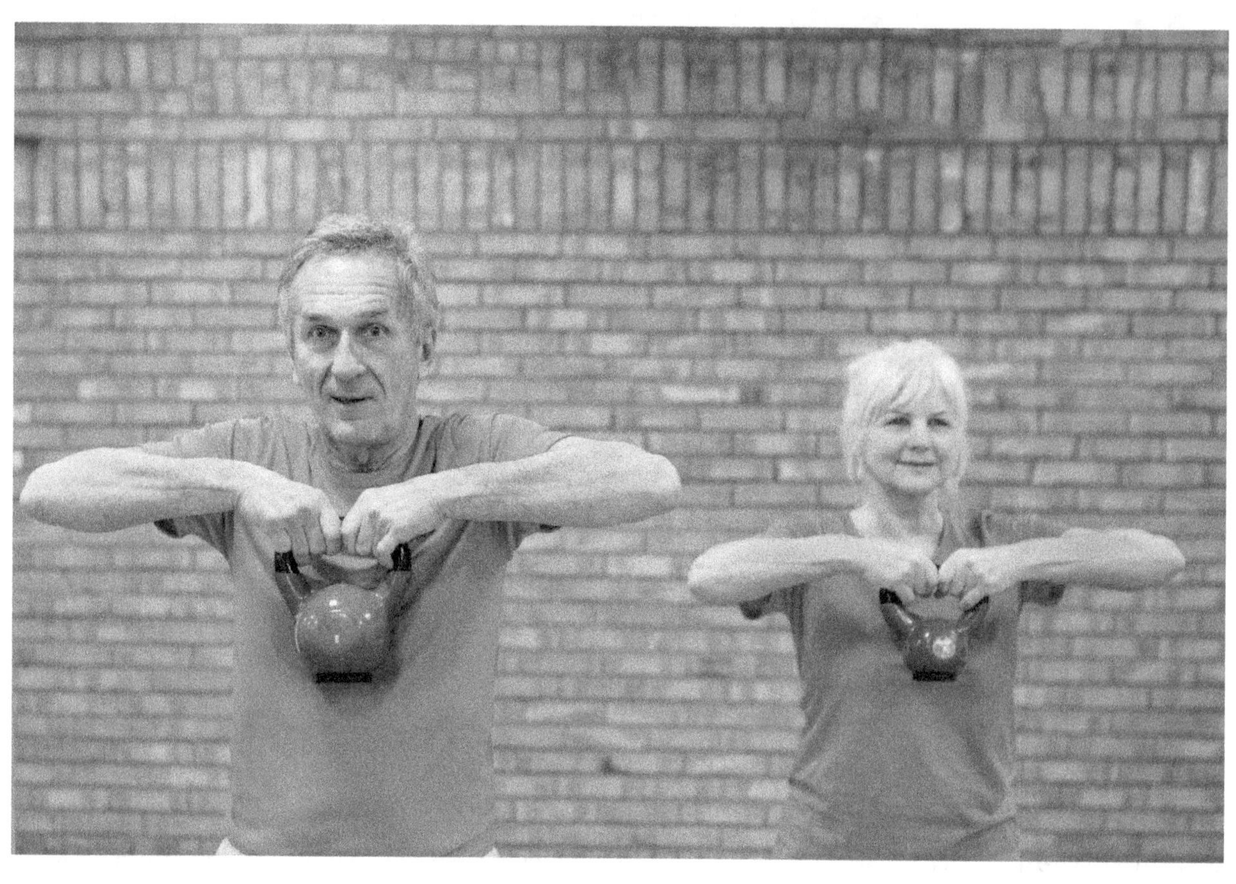

<u>Chapter 2: The Power of 5 Minutes</u>

In this chapter, we will explore the significance of incorporating short but consistent exercise sessions into the daily routine of seniors. Discover how just five minutes of exercise can make a positive impact on physical and mental well-being.

1. <u>The Concept of Five-Minute Exercise:</u>

a. Briefly explain the concept of five-minute exercise.
b. Emphasize the simplicity and accessibility of incorporating short exercise sessions into daily life.

2. <u>Physical Health Benefits:</u>

a. Highlight the physical health benefits of five-minute exercise sessions.
i. Improved cardiovascular health and circulation.
ii. Increased strength and flexibility.
iii. Enhanced balance and coordination.
iv. Reduced risk of chronic diseases.

3. <u>Mental Health Benefits:</u>

a. Showcase the mental health benefits of five-minute exercise sessions.

i. Reduced stress and anxiety.
ii. Improved mood and happiness.
iii. Enhanced cognitive function and memory.
iv. Increased self-confidence and self-esteem.

4. <u>Practical Ideas for Five-Minute Exercises:</u>

a. Provide a variety of practical ideas for five-minute exercises that seniors can engage in.

i. Gentle stretching routines.
ii. Short walks or light aerobic exercises.
iii. Balance and stability exercises.
iv. Chair-based exercises for those with limited mobility.

5. Overcoming Barriers:
a. Address common barriers that seniors might encounter when adopting a five-minute exercise routine.
i. Lack of motivation or time.
ii. Physical limitations or chronic conditions.
iii. Fear of injury or discomfort.
iv. Lack of social support or encouragement.

6. Tips for Success:
a. Offer practical tips to help seniors succeed in incorporating five-minute exercise sessions into their routine.
i. Set achievable goals and gradually increase exercise duration.
ii. Find a form of exercise that is enjoyable and fits personal preferences.
iii. Seek support from family, friends, or exercise groups.
iv. Track progress and celebrate small victories.

Reiterate the power of five-minute exercise and the significant positive impact it can have on the physical and mental well-being of seniors. Encourage readers to embrace these short exercise sessions as a simple yet effective way to enhance their overall quality of life.

Disclaimer: Always consult with a healthcare professional before starting any new exercise program to ensure it is safe and suitable for your individual needs.

A. <u>Explaining the concept of short and effective workouts</u>

Short and effective workouts are an approach to exercise that focuses on maximizing the benefits within a limited timeframe. The concept recognizes that not everyone has hours to dedicate to lengthy gym sessions or workouts, and instead, it emphasizes the efficiency of shorter bursts of exercise.

<u>The key principles of short and effective workouts are:</u>

1. High Intensity:
Short workouts often involve high-intensity exercises that challenge your body and get your heart rate up quickly. By pushing yourself to work harder in a shorter amount of time, you can achieve similar or even greater results compared to longer, lower-intensity workouts.

2. Compound Movements:
These workouts typically incorporate compound movements that engage multiple muscle groups simultaneously. Exercises like squats, lunges, push-ups, and burpees are examples of compound movements that provide a full-body workout and maximize calorie burn.

3. Interval Training:
Interval training involves alternating between periods of intense exercise and short recovery periods. This approach helps to increase cardiovascular fitness, burn more calories, and improve endurance within a shorter timeframe.

4. Circuit Training:
Circuit training involves performing a series of exercises one after another, or in a specific circuit, with minimal rest periods in between. This keeps your heart rate elevated and targets different muscle groups, providing a comprehensive workout in a shorter duration.

5. Functional Movements:
Short workouts often focus on functional movements that mimic everyday activities or sports-specific motions. These movements improve strength, flexibility, and coordination, making activities of daily living easier and reducing the risk of injury.

<u>Benefits of Short and Effective Workouts:</u>

1. Time Efficiency:

Short workouts are ideal for individuals with busy schedules as they require less time commitment. It allows you to fit exercise into your day without sacrificing other responsibilities.

2. Increased Fat Burning:
High-intensity exercises and interval training stimulate your metabolism and help burn more calories during and after the workout. This can be especially beneficial for weight loss or weight maintenance goals.

3. Improved Fitness Levels:
Short and effective workouts challenge your cardiovascular system, build strength, and enhance endurance. Regular practice can lead to improved overall fitness and athletic performance.

4. Convenience and Accessibility:
Short workouts can be done with minimal equipment and in various settings, such as at home, in a park, or while traveling. This makes it easier to maintain an exercise routine regardless of location or circumstances.

5. Motivation and Variety:
For individuals who find longer workouts monotonous or struggle with motivation, short and varied workouts can be more appealing. It allows for flexibility in trying different exercises and keeping the workout routine fresh and engaging.

Remember to listen to your body, warm up adequately, and consult with a healthcare professional before starting any new exercise program, especially if you have any underlying health conditions or concerns.

B. <u>Benefits of incorporating brief exercise sessions into daily routine</u>

Incorporating brief exercise sessions into your daily routine offers several benefits for your physical and mental well-being. Here are some key advantages:

1. _Increased Energy Levels_:

Engaging in short exercise sessions can provide a quick boost of energy and help combat feelings of fatigue or sluggishness throughout the day.

2. Improved Physical Fitness:
Even brief exercise sessions can contribute to improved physical fitness. Regular activity, even in short bursts, can help strengthen muscles, improve cardiovascular health, and enhance flexibility and endurance.

3. Weight Management:
Incorporating brief exercise sessions into your daily routine can support weight management efforts. Regular physical activity helps to burn calories, increase metabolism, and maintain a healthy body composition.

4. Mental Clarity and Focus:
Short exercise sessions have been shown to enhance cognitive function, including improved focus, concentration, and mental clarity. Physical activity stimulates the brain, promoting better productivity and mental performance.

5. Mood Enhancement:
Exercise releases endorphins, commonly known as "feel-good" hormones. Even short bursts of exercise can trigger the release of these hormones, contributing to improved mood, reduced stress levels, and increased overall well-being.

6. Better Sleep Quality:
Regular exercise, even in shorter durations, can improve sleep quality and duration. Engaging in physical activity during the day helps regulate the sleep-wake cycle, promoting a more restful and rejuvenating sleep at night.

7. Reduced Risk of Chronic Diseases:
Consistent participation in brief exercise sessions can help reduce the risk of chronic diseases such as heart disease, high blood pressure, type 2 diabetes, and certain types of cancer.

8. Time Management:

Short exercise sessions are ideal for those with busy schedules or limited time. By incorporating brief workouts into your routine, you can prioritize your health and fitness without disrupting other responsibilities and commitments.

9. Sustainable Approach:
Incorporating brief exercise sessions into your daily routine is a sustainable approach to maintaining an active lifestyle. It requires less time commitment, reducing the likelihood of burnout or feeling overwhelmed by lengthy workouts.

10. Long-Term Health Benefits:
Consistency is key when it comes to exercise. By integrating short exercise sessions into your daily routine, you establish a habit of regular physical activity, leading to long-term health benefits and a reduced risk of age-related health concerns.

Remember, a combination of strength, flexibility, cardiovascular, and balance exercises is ideal for a well-rounded fitness routine. Consult with a healthcare professional or fitness expert to determine the most appropriate exercises for your individual needs and capabilities.

C. <u>Overcoming barriers to exercise through 5-minute workouts</u>

Overcoming barriers to exercise is an important aspect of adopting a regular fitness routine. Incorporating 5-minute workouts can be particularly helpful in overcoming these barriers. Here's how:

1. Lack of Time:
Many individuals struggle to find time for exercise due to busy schedules. 5-minute workouts provide a practical solution by requiring minimal time commitment. They can be easily squeezed into breaks throughout the day, such as during work breaks or before meal preparation.

2. Lack of Motivation:
Finding motivation to exercise can be challenging, especially when longer workouts seem overwhelming. 5-minute workouts offer a manageable goal

that feels less daunting. By starting with short bursts of activity, you can gain momentum and gradually increase your motivation to exercise.

3. Physical Limitations or Chronic Conditions:
Some individuals may have physical limitations or chronic conditions that make traditional workout routines difficult. 5-minute workouts can be customized to accommodate these limitations. Focus on exercises that are gentle, low-impact, and suited to your abilities. Chair exercises or modified movements can be great options.

4. Lack of Equipment or Space:
Traditional workouts often require specialized equipment or ample space, which may not be readily available. 5-minute workouts can be designed using bodyweight exercises or simple props like resistance bands or small weights. They can be performed anywhere, such as in a small room, office, or even outdoors.

5. Intimidation or Discomfort:
Starting a new exercise routine can be intimidating, especially if you're unsure about proper form or worried about feeling uncomfortable in a gym setting. 5-minute workouts offer a non-intimidating and private option. You can perform them in the comfort of your own home, ensuring a judgment-free environment.

6. Lack of Variety:
Doing the same exercises repeatedly can lead to workout boredom. With 5-minute workouts, you have the opportunity to vary the exercises every day or focus on different muscle groups. This variety keeps your routine interesting and enjoyable.

7. Social Support:
Some individuals may lack social support or exercise buddies, which can make it harder to stay motivated. Engaging in 5-minute workouts allows you to connect with online fitness communities or seek virtual support from friends and family. Sharing progress and achievements can provide the necessary encouragement to keep going.

Remember, the key to making 5-minute workouts effective is to ensure that exercises are performed safely and with proper form. If needed, consult with a healthcare professional or a fitness instructor to determine appropriate exercises for your specific needs and goals.

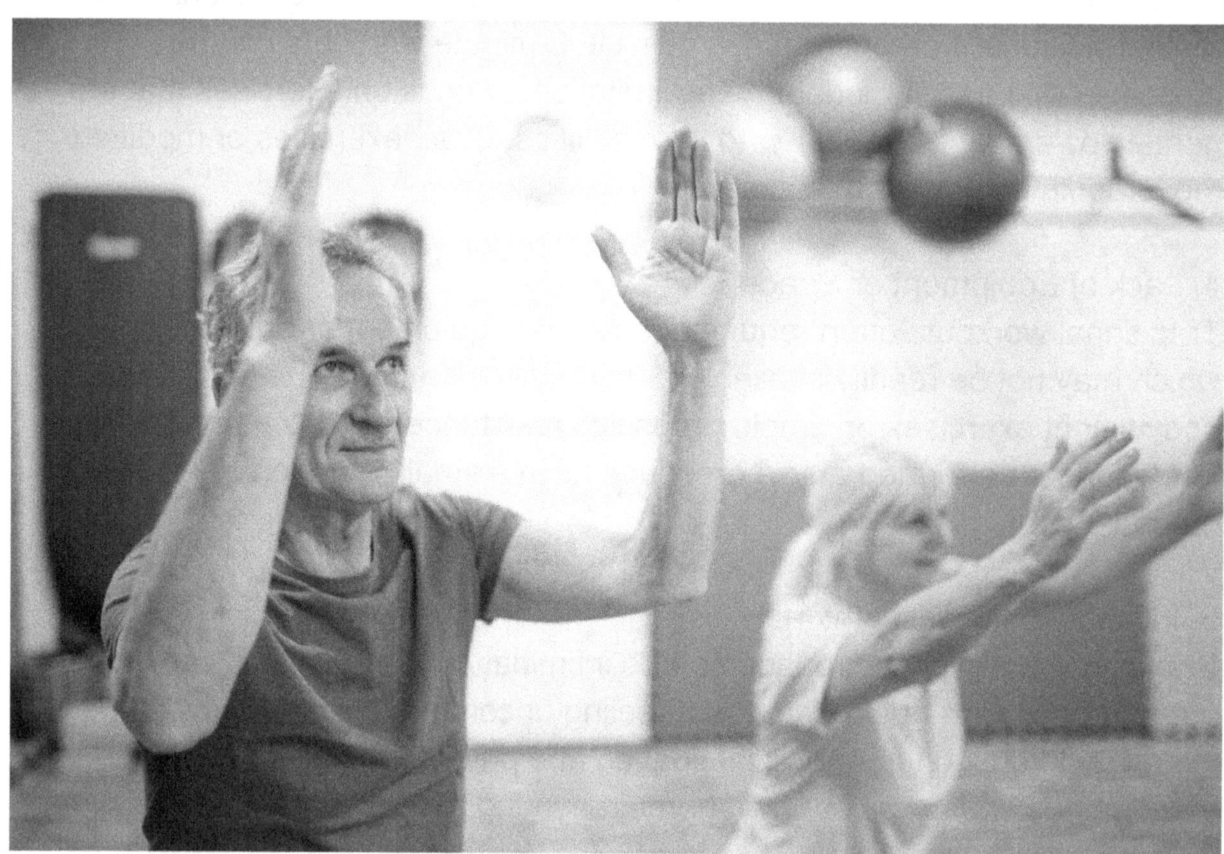

Chapter 3: The Essential Components of a 5-Minute Fitness Routine

In this chapter, we will explore the essential components that make up an effective 5-minute fitness routine specifically designed for senior citizens. These components are designed to improve strength, flexibility, balance, and overall well-being. By incorporating these exercises into your daily routine, you can maintain an active and healthy lifestyle.

1. Warm-Up Exercises:
Before starting any exercise routine, it's crucial to warm up your muscles and prepare your body for physical activity. The warm-up exercises are aimed at increasing blood flow, raising body temperature, and loosening the joints. Some simple warm-up exercises for seniors include:
- Shoulder rolls
- Neck stretches
- Ankle circles
- Arm swings
- Marching in place

2. Aerobic Exercises:
Aerobic exercises are essential for cardiovascular health and overall fitness. These exercises increase heart rate, improve stamina, and boost lung capacity. Some low-impact aerobic exercises suitable for seniors include:
- Brisk walking
- Cycling
- Water aerobics
- Dancing
- Chair exercises

3. Strength Training:
Strength training is crucial for maintaining muscle mass, improving bone density, and increasing overall strength. While it's important to start with lightweight or no weights, gradually increasing resistance can gradually build strength over time. Some strength exercises for seniors include:

- Squats
- Wall push-ups
- Leg lifts
- Bicep curls with dumbbells
- Resistance band exercises

4. Flexibility Exercises:
Flexibility exercises help maintain joint mobility, improve posture, and prevent injuries. Stretching exercises performed regularly can increase flexibility, reduce stiffness, and enhance overall mobility. Some flexibility exercises for seniors include:
- Neck stretches
- Shoulder and chest stretches
- Hamstring stretches
- Quadriceps stretches
- Calf stretches

5. Balance and Stability Exercises:
Balance exercises are crucial for preventing falls and maintaining stability. These exercises help strengthen the muscles responsible for balance, improve coordination, and build confidence. Some balance exercises for seniors include:
- Heel-to-toe walk
- Single-leg stands
- Yoga poses like Tree Pose or Warrior Pose
- Tai Chi exercises
- Standing leg lifts

Incorporating these essential components into a 5-minute fitness routine for senior citizens can have significant benefits on overall health and well-being. Remember to consult with a healthcare professional before starting any new exercise program, especially if you have any underlying health conditions. Regular physical activity is key to maintaining a healthy and active lifestyle, and even a short routine can make a big difference.

B. <u>Low-impact cardio exercises</u>

Low-impact cardio exercises are beneficial for senior citizens as they provide cardiovascular benefits without putting too much strain on the joints. Here are some examples of low-impact cardio exercises suitable for seniors:

1. Brisk Walking: Take a brisk walk either outdoors or on a treadmill. Start with a comfortable pace and gradually increase the speed over time. Aim for at least 10-15 minutes of brisk walking.

2. Cycling: Whether it's on a stationary bike or a regular bicycle, cycling is a low-impact exercise that strengthens the legs and improves cardiovascular fitness. Start with shorter durations and gradually increase the duration as you become more comfortable.

3. Water Aerobics: Joining a water aerobics class or performing exercises in a pool is a great way to get a low-impact cardio workout. The water provides resistance and support, making it easier on the joints. Perform exercises such as water walking, leg kicks, or arm movements in the water.

4. Dancing: Dancing is a fun and engaging low-impact cardio exercise. Choose dance styles that are gentle on the joints, such as ballroom dancing or low-impact aerobic dance classes. You can dance around in your living room or join a dance class specifically designed for seniors.

5. Chair Exercises: If mobility is limited, chair exercises can be an excellent option for low-impact cardio. Perform exercises like seated marching, chair boxing, or seated leg extensions. These exercises can elevate the heart rate while seated and provide a cardio workout.

Remember to start slowly and gradually increase intensity and duration as your fitness level improves. It's essential to listen to your body and not overexert yourself. Always consult with a healthcare professional before starting any new exercise program to ensure it aligns with your specific needs and medical conditions.

C. <u>Strength training exercises</u>

Strength training exercises are essential for seniors as they help maintain muscle mass, improve bone density, and increase overall strength. Here are some strength training exercises suitable for senior citizens:

1. Squats:
Stand with your feet shoulder-width apart. Slowly lower your body as if you are sitting back in a chair, keeping your chest up and your knees aligned with your toes. Aim to lower until your thighs are parallel to the floor, and then push through your heels to stand back up. Start with a chair behind you for support, if necessary.

2. Wall Push-Ups:
Stand facing a wall, about an arm's length away. Place your hands on the wall at shoulder height and slightly wider than shoulder width apart. Lean forward, bending your elbows, and bring your chest closer to the wall. Push back to the starting position. Adjust the distance from the wall to make it easier or harder, depending on your strength.

3. Leg Lifts:
Stand behind a chair or hold onto a countertop for support. Lift one leg straight back while keeping your back straight and your core engaged. Hold for a moment, then slowly lower the leg back down. Repeat with the other leg. This exercise strengthens the muscles in your buttocks and the back of your thighs.

4. Bicep Curls with Dumbbells:
Hold a dumbbell in each hand, palms facing forward. Keep your back straight and your elbows close to your sides. Bend your elbows and bring the dumbbells up towards your shoulders, contracting your bicep muscles. Lower the dumbbells back down to the starting position. Start with lighter weights and gradually increase as you feel comfortable.

5. Resistance Band Exercises:
Resistance bands provide a gentle and effective way to build strength. Sit on a chair with the band securely under your feet. Hold the ends of the band in

your hands, palms facing upward. Slowly curl your hands towards your shoulders, bending at the elbows. Gradually release the tension and return to the starting position. You can perform various exercises with resistance bands, targeting different muscle groups.

Remember to start with lighter weights or resistance and gradually increase as your strength improves. Perform each exercise with proper form and control. It's always recommended to consult with a healthcare professional or a certified fitness trainer before starting any new exercise program, especially if you have underlying health conditions.

D. <u>Flexibility and balance exercises</u>

Flexibility and balance exercises are vital for senior citizens as they help maintain joint mobility, improve posture, and prevent falls. Here are some examples of flexibility and balance exercises suitable for seniors:

1. Neck Stretches:
Sit or stand tall, and slowly tilt your head to the right, bringing your right ear towards your right shoulder. Hold for a few seconds, then repeat on the left side. Do this stretch a few times on each side.

2. Shoulder and Chest Stretches:
Stand with your feet shoulder-width apart. Extend one arm across your chest and gently pull it towards your opposite shoulder. Hold for a few seconds, then switch to the other arm. Repeat several times on each side.

3. Hamstring Stretches:
Sit on the edge of a chair with one leg extended straight out in front of you. Gently lean forward, reaching towards your toes while keeping your back straight. Hold for a few seconds, then switch legs. Repeat a few times on each leg.

4. Quadriceps Stretches:
Stand near a wall or a chair for support. Bend one knee and reach back to grab your ankle or foot with the hand on the same side. Gently pull your foot

towards your buttocks, feeling a stretch in the front of your thigh. Hold for a few seconds, then switch legs. Repeat a few times on each leg.

5. Calf Stretches:
Stand facing a wall and place your hands on the wall for support. Step one foot back, keeping it straight with the heel on the ground. Bend your front knee while keeping the back leg extended, feeling a stretch in your calf muscle. Hold for a few seconds, then switch legs. Repeat a few times on each leg.

<u>Balance Exercises:</u>

1. Heel-to-Toe Walk:
Position your heel to touch the toes of the opposite foot, walk in a straight line. Take small, deliberate steps, placing your heel directly in front of the toes of the other foot with each step. Repeat for a short distance or time.

2. Single-Leg Stands:
Stand beside a chair or wall for support. Lift one foot off the ground and balance on the other foot. Hold this position for 20-30 seconds, then switch feet. As you get more comfortable, try to balance without any support.

3. Yoga Poses:
Certain yoga poses can help improve balance and flexibility. Tree Pose and Warrior Pose are two examples that can be modified for seniors. Practice these poses with proper guidance and support.

4. Tai Chi Exercises:
Tai Chi incorporates slow, flowing movements that improve balance and coordination. Joining a Tai Chi class specifically designed for seniors can be beneficial to learn and practice the exercises correctly.

5. Standing Leg Lifts:
Stand behind a chair for support. Slowly lift one leg straight out to the side, keeping it straight or with a slight bend at the knee. Hold the position for a few seconds, then lower the leg. Repeat with the other leg. Perform several repetitions on each leg.

Remember to perform these exercises in a controlled manner and breathe deeply throughout. Modify or adjust exercises as needed based on your comfort level and abilities. Always consult with a healthcare professional or a certified fitness trainer before starting any new exercise program.

E. <u>Cool-down and stretching exercises</u>

Cool-down and stretching exercises are essential for seniors to gradually bring down their heart rate and relax the muscles after physical activity. Here are some cool-down and stretching exercises suitable for senior citizens:

1. Slow Walking:
After completing your exercise session, gradually decrease the intensity of your movement by walking slowly for a few minutes. This helps bring your heart rate down gradually.

2. Arm Swings:
Stand with your feet shoulder-width apart and let your arms hang loosely at your sides. Slowly swing your arms forward and backward in a controlled motion for 10-15 seconds. This helps loosen up the shoulder and arm muscles.

3. Gentle Stretching:
Perform gentle stretches for the major muscle groups you targeted during your exercise routine. Take slow, deep breaths while holding each stretch for 15-30 seconds. Focus on the areas such as the calves, thighs, hips, chest, shoulders, and arms.

<u>Stretching Exercises:</u>

1. Calf Stretch:
Stand facing a wall, about arm's length away. Place your hands on the wall for support. Step one foot forward and bend the knee, keeping the back leg straight with the heel on the ground. Lean forward until you feel a gentle stretch in your calf. Hold for 15-30 seconds, then switch legs.

2. Quadriceps Stretch:
Stand near a wall or a chair for support. Bend one knee and grab your ankle or foot with the hand on the same side. Gently pull your foot towards your buttocks, feeling a stretch in the front of your thigh. Hold for 15-30 seconds, then switch legs.

3. Triceps Stretch:
Extend one arm overhead, reaching towards the opposite side. Bend the elbow and let your hand drop behind your head. With your other hand, reach behind your back and try to grasp your fingers or hold onto a towel. Hold for 15-30 seconds, then switch sides.

4. Chest Stretch:
Stand tall with your feet shoulder-width apart. Clasp your hands behind your back, with your arms straight. Gently lift your arms backward while squeezing your shoulder blades together. Hold for 15-30 seconds.

5. Shoulder Rolls:
Stand with your feet shoulder-width apart. Roll your shoulders forward in a circular motion, gradually increasing the range of motion. After a few seconds, reverse the motion and roll your shoulders backward. Repeat a few times in each direction.

Remember to stretch gently and avoid forcing any movement. If you feel any pain or discomfort, ease off the stretch. It's important to listen to your body and never push beyond your limits. If you have any underlying health conditions or concerns, consult with a healthcare professional before starting any new exercise program.

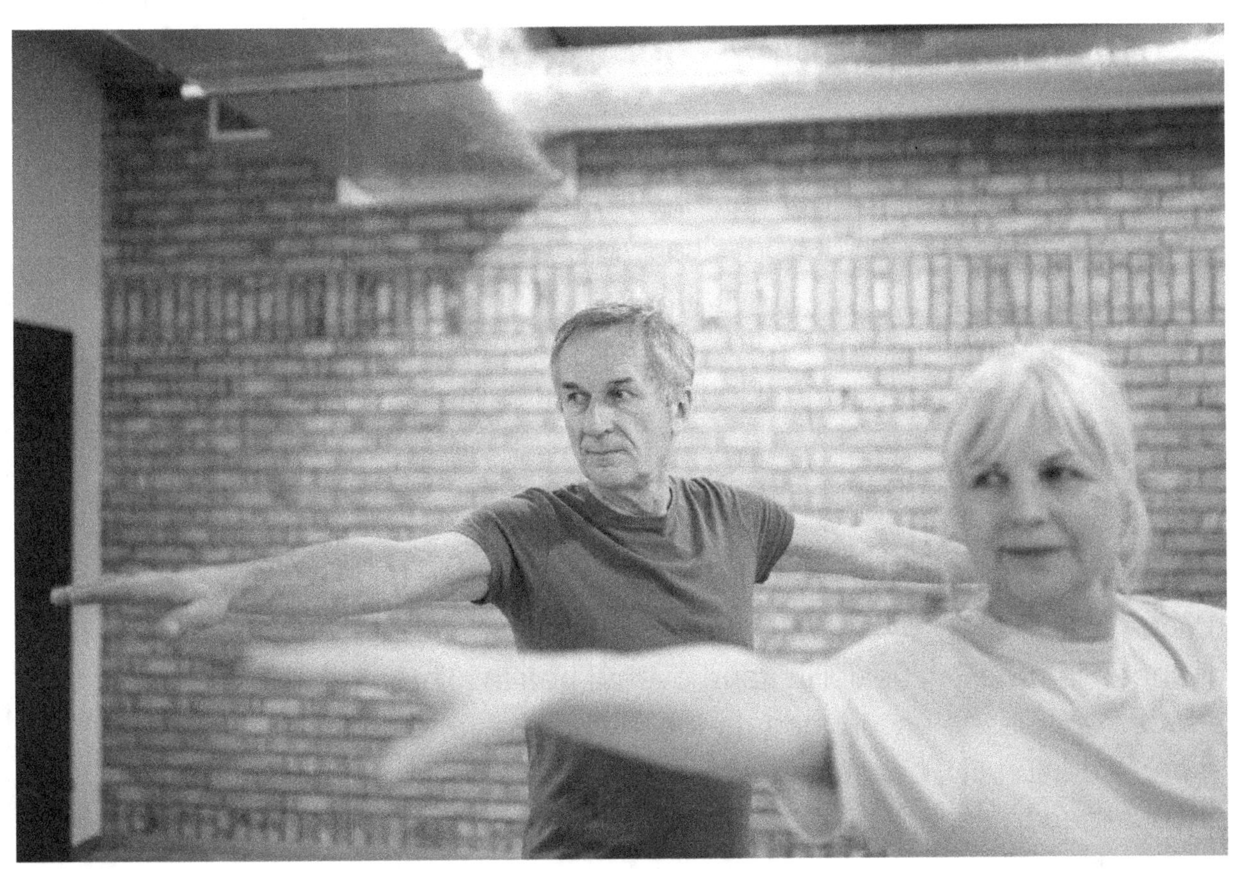

<u>Chapter 4: Tailoring Your 5-Minute Fitness Routine</u>

Chapter 4 of our book will discuss the importance of tailoring your 5-minute fitness routine specifically for senior citizens. As we age, it becomes even more crucial to prioritize our physical well-being and incorporate regular exercise into our daily lives. This chapter will provide you with valuable insights and guidance on how to create a personalized and effective fitness routine to suit the needs and capabilities of senior citizens.

<u>Understanding the Unique Needs of Senior Citizens:</u>

Before delving into creating a fitness routine, it's essential to understand the unique needs and considerations of senior citizens. Aging often brings about changes in mobility, flexibility, and overall health. Therefore, it's important to adapt exercises to accommodate these changes and minimize the risk of injury. Additionally, consulting with a healthcare professional is highly encouraged to ensure that the chosen exercises are safe for individual circumstances.

<u>Creating a Tailored 5-Minute Fitness Routine:</u>

Here are some key considerations and steps to create a personalized 5-minute fitness routine for senior citizens:

1. Warm-up:
Begin your routine with a gentle warm-up to prepare the body for exercise. This could include light stretching or range-of-motion exercises to increase flexibility and promote blood flow.

2. Strength Exercises:
Incorporate strength exercises that target major muscle groups. These exercises help maintain muscle mass, improve bone density, and enhance overall strength. Simple activities like chair squats, leg lifts, or resistance band exercises can be effective and safe for seniors.

3. Balance and Coordination:

To improve balance and coordination, include exercises specifically designed for these areas. This could involve standing on one leg, heel-to-toe walks, or practicing tai chi movements. Enhancing balance can significantly reduce the risk of falls, which is a common concern among seniors.

4. Cardiovascular Activities:
Engaging in cardiovascular exercises can benefit heart health and overall fitness. For seniors, low-impact activities like walking, swimming, or cycling are highly recommended. These exercises are gentle on the joints and can be customized based on individual fitness levels and capabilities.

5. Flexibility and Stretching:
Promote flexibility and joint mobility through specific stretches and flexibility exercises. Stretching the major muscle groups can help maintain range of motion, reduce muscle stiffness, and enhance overall flexibility.

In this chapter, we have explored the significance of tailoring a 5-minute fitness routine specifically for senior citizens. By understanding their unique needs and limitations, we can create a safe and effective workout plan that promotes physical well-being. Remember to consult with a healthcare professional and consider individual abilities and requirements when designing a fitness routine for seniors.

Disclaimer: It is always recommended to consult with a healthcare professional before starting any exercise program, especially for senior citizens.

A. For those people who will be creating a program for seniors.

Understanding individual senior citizens' fitness levels and limitations is crucial when tailoring a fitness routine for them. Here are some ways to assess and gather information about their abilities:

1. Consultation with Healthcare Professional:
Encourage seniors to consult with their healthcare provider, such as a physician or physical therapist, who can assess their overall health, mobility,

and any specific limitations or conditions that need to be considered in their fitness routine.

2. Health History and Medical Conditions:
Ask seniors about their health history and any current medical conditions, such as arthritis, osteoporosis, cardiovascular issues, or joint problems. Understanding these factors will help determine which exercises are safe and appropriate for them.

3. Physical Assessments:
Conduct simple physical assessments to evaluate strength, balance, and flexibility. For example, observe their ability to stand up from a chair without assistance or maintain balance while performing certain movements. These assessments can provide insights into their current fitness level and functional abilities.

4. Communication and Feedback:
Engage in open and honest communication with the seniors, encouraging them to share their experiences, concerns, and any discomfort they may feel during physical activity. Regularly ask for feedback to make adjustments to the routine as necessary.

5. Progression and Adaptation:
As seniors become more comfortable with their routine, continue to monitor their progress, and adjust the exercises accordingly. Gradually increase the intensity or duration of exercises or introduce new activities to challenge them and prevent plateaus.

Remember, every senior citizen is unique, and their fitness levels and limitations may vary. By understanding and addressing their individual needs, you can create a tailored fitness routine that promotes their overall well-being and helps them achieve their fitness goals.

B. <u>Modifying exercises to suit specific needs and abilities</u>

Modifying exercises to suit specific senior citizens' needs and abilities is essential to ensure their safety and progress. Here are some guidelines to consider when adapting exercises for seniors:

1. Individual Assessment:
Assess each senior's abilities, limitations, and fitness level before designing their exercise program. Consider factors such as strength, balance, flexibility, mobility, and any existing medical conditions or injuries. This will help you understand their specific needs and determine suitable modifications.

2. Exercise Selection:
Choose exercises that are appropriate for the individual's abilities and goals. Opt for low-impact activities that minimize strain on joints and consider exercises that target specific areas needing improvement, such as strength, balance, or flexibility.

3. Reduce Impact and Joint Stress:
Modify exercises to reduce the impact on joints and minimize the risk of injury. For example, instead of high-impact movements like jumping jacks, consider low-impact alternatives like marching in place or seated knee lifts.

4. Decrease Range of Motion:
If a senior has a limited range of motion, you can modify exercises by reducing the range of motion required. For instance, instead of a full squat, they can perform a partial squat or use a chair for support.

5. Use Supportive Equipment:
Utilize supportive equipment to assist seniors during exercises. This may include stability balls, resistance bands, or chairs for balance and support. Such equipment can make exercises more accessible and safe for individuals with compromised stability or strength.

6. Adjust Intensity:
Modify the intensity of exercises based on the individual's fitness level. This can be done by manipulating factors such as repetitions, duration, resistance,

or the speed of movements. Gradually increase these factors as their fitness improves.

7. Provide Options for Different Abilities:
Offer variations or options for exercises to accommodate different abilities within a group of senior citizens. This allows individuals to choose the level of difficulty that suits them best and fosters inclusivity in the fitness routine.

8. Incorporate Rest Periods:
Allow sufficient rest periods during the workout to prevent excessive fatigue and ensure the senior can maintain proper form throughout the session. Encourage participants to listen to their bodies and rest as needed.

9. Regular Communication and Feedback:
Maintain open communication with seniors to ensure that exercises are comfortable, appropriate, and effective for them. Encourage them to provide feedback on any discomfort or difficulties experienced during the workout, so modifications can be made if necessary.

Remember, individualizing exercises for senior citizens is key to their safety and overall progress. By adapting exercises to their abilities and needs, you can create a more inclusive and beneficial fitness routine for them.

C. <u>Remember to adapt the routines as fitness improves</u>

As a senior citizen's fitness improves, it is important to adapt their fitness routine to continue challenging them and promoting further progress. Here are some strategies for modifying the routine as a senior's fitness improves:

1. Increase Intensity:
Gradually increase the intensity of exercises to provide a greater challenge. This can be accomplished by adding resistance, increasing repetitions or sets, or performing exercises at a faster pace. For example, if a senior is comfortable with bodyweight squats, you can introduce weighted squats or lunges to increase the resistance.

2. Add Variety:
Introduce new exercises or variations of existing exercises to engage different muscle groups and prevent boredom. This can also help seniors continue to improve their overall fitness by targeting different areas. For example, if they have been primarily focusing on lower body exercises, incorporate upper body exercises like bicep curls or overhead presses.

3. Progress Range of Motion:
As seniors become more flexible and mobile, gradually increase the range of motion in exercises. This can be done by encouraging them to deepen their squats or lunges, extend their stretches further, or gradually increase the range of motion in joint movements. However, it is crucial to monitor their form and ensure they maintain proper technique throughout.

4. Challenge Balance and Stability:
As balance and stability improve, incorporate exercises that challenge these aspects further. This can include performing single-leg exercises like single-leg balances or single-leg deadlifts. Incorporating balance-oriented activities like yoga or tai chi can also be beneficial.

5. Shorten Rest Periods:
As seniors progress, they may be able to reduce their rest periods between exercises. Shortening the rest periods helps to maintain an elevated heart rate and improves cardiovascular fitness. However, it is important to strike a balance and ensure they have enough recovery time to perform exercises with proper form and prevent overexertion.

6. Set New Goals:
Continually set new goals with seniors as their fitness improves. This can help maintain their motivation and focus on their continued progress. Encourage them to strive for specific achievements, such as increasing the number of repetitions or holding a balance pose for a longer duration.

7. Monitor and Adjust:
Continuously monitor the senior's progress and listen to their feedback. Adjust the routine as needed based on their capabilities, comfort level, and any

changes in their health or physical condition. Regularly communicate with them to ensure the routine remains challenging but manageable.

Adapting the routine as a senior's fitness improves is essential to prevent plateaus and promote ongoing progress. By gradually increasing intensity, adding variety, and setting new goals, seniors can continue to improve their physical fitness and overall well-being.

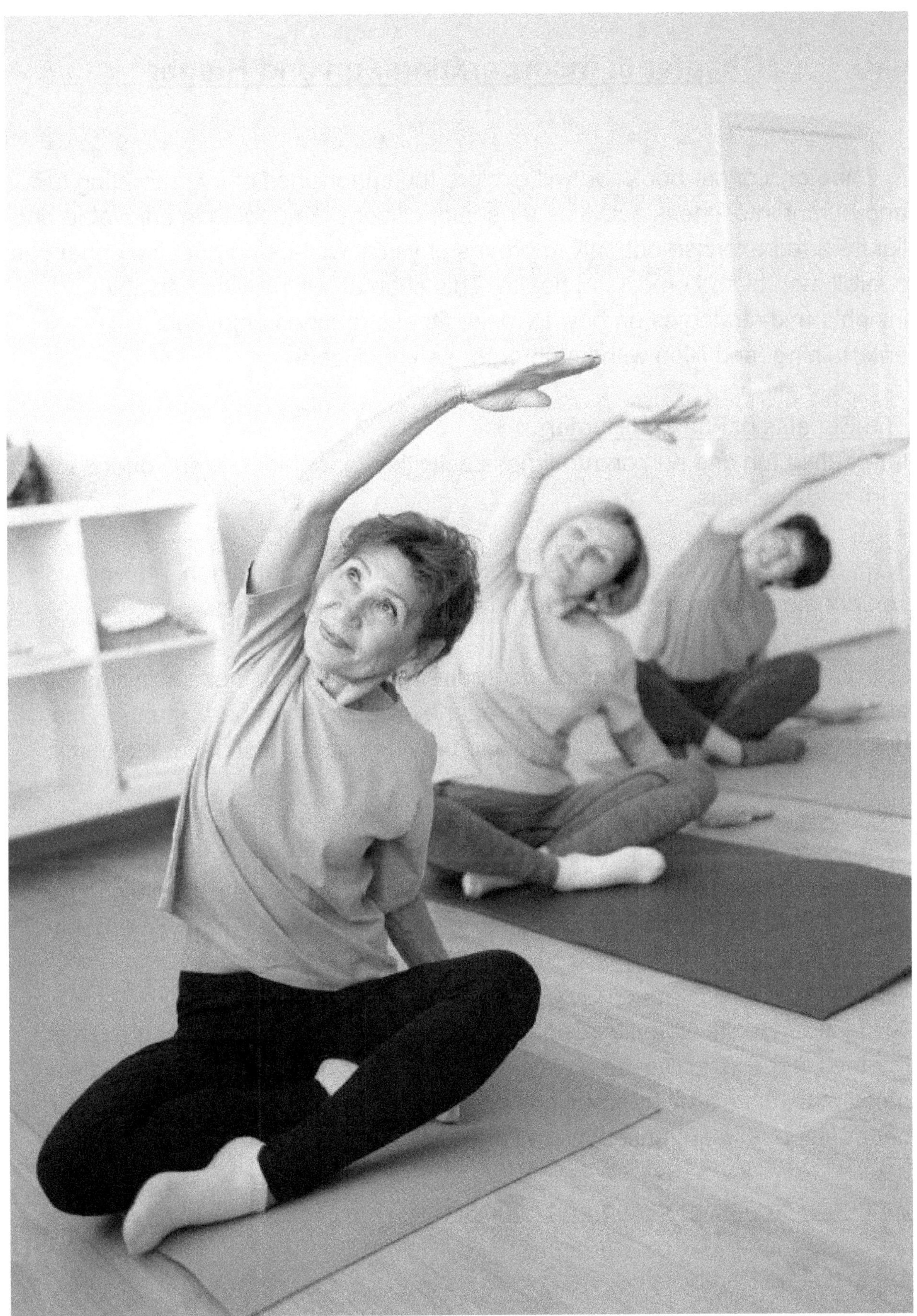

Chapter 5: Incorporating Fun and Humor

In Chapter 5 of our book, we will explore the importance of incorporating fun and humor into fitness activities for senior citizens. Engaging in enjoyable and lighthearted exercise not only improves physical well-being but also enhances overall mental and emotional health. This chapter will provide valuable insights and strategies on how to make fitness routines enjoyable, entertaining, and filled with laughter for senior citizens.

<u>The Benefits of Fun and Humor:</u>
Integrating fun and humor into fitness activities for senior citizens offers numerous benefits:

1. Increased Motivation: Fun and laughter can boost motivation, making seniors more eager to participate in regular exercise routines.

2. Enhanced Social Interaction: Incorporating enjoyable fitness activities encourages socialization and camaraderie among senior participants. This helps foster a sense of community and provides opportunities for friendship and connection.

3. Improved Mental Well-being: Laughter and fun release endorphins, reducing stress levels and improving overall mental well-being. This can help combat anxiety, depression, and other mental health challenges commonly faced by seniors.

4. Physical Health Benefits: Engaging in enjoyable and entertaining exercise routines leads to increased physical activity levels. Regular physical activity helps maintain a healthy weight, improves cardiovascular health, promotes better sleep, and enhances overall physical fitness.

<u>Strategies for Incorporating Fun and Humor:</u>

1. Music and Dance:

Play upbeat music during exercise sessions and encourage seniors to move to the rhythm. Incorporate dance movements or simple choreography to make it more enjoyable. Remember to select music that resonates with the participants' preferences and offers a nostalgic touch.

2. Games and Challenges:

Introduce games and challenges that incorporate exercise. For instance, set up a friendly competition involving target throwing, relay races, or balloon volleyball. These activities add an element of fun, friendly rivalry, and excitement to the routine.

3. Theme-based Workouts:

Organize theme-based workouts where participants dress up or focus on a particular era, such as the 60s or 70s. Design exercises and movements that align with the chosen theme to make the routine more entertaining and engaging.

4. Humor and Jokes:

Incorporate humor and jokes into the fitness session to lighten the atmosphere. Share lighthearted jokes, humorous anecdotes, or funny stories during breaks or transitions. Laughter can enhance the enjoyment and leave participants feeling happy and energized.

5. Props and Accessories:

Utilize props and accessories to add an element of playfulness and creativity to the exercises. For example, use colorful exercise balls, resistance bands, or scarves to make movements more engaging and enjoyable. Encourage seniors to embrace their inner child and have fun with these props.

6. Recreational Activities:

Incorporate recreational activities such as nature walks, gardening, or outdoor games to make fitness a part of an enjoyable and leisurely experience. Being in a natural setting can enhance the enjoyment of the exercise routine and provide additional mental and emotional benefits.

In this chapter, we have highlighted the importance of incorporating fun and humor into fitness activities for senior citizens. By making exercise enjoyable and entertaining, we can effectively motivate seniors to participate regularly and experience the physical, mental, and social benefits. Remember, laughter is the best medicine, so let's keep fitness routines for seniors filled with fun and joy!

A. The Role of Laughter in Promoting Wellness

Laughter plays a vital role in promoting wellness for senior citizens. Here's how laughter benefits their overall well-being:

1. Physical Benefits:

a. Boosts Immune System: Laughter increases the production of antibodies and activates immune cells, strengthening the immune system and helping seniors stay healthier.
b. Relieves Pain: Laughing triggers the release of endorphins, natural painkillers that can provide temporary relief from physical discomfort.
c. Increases Blood Flow: Laughing improves blood vessel function, enhancing blood flow and oxygenation to the body's organs and tissues.

2. Mental and Emotional Benefits:

a. Reduces Stress: Laughter reduces the production of stress hormones, such as cortisol, and stimulates the release of feel-good hormones, promoting a sense of relaxation and well-being.
b. Improves Mood: Seniors who engage in regular laughter often experience improved mood and decreased feelings of depression and anxiety.
c. Enhances Cognitive Function: Laughter stimulates brain activity, promoting mental alertness, memory, and overall cognitive function.

3. Social Benefits:

a. Enhances Social Connection: Laughing together fosters a sense of camaraderie and social bonding among seniors. It can strengthen relationships, reduce feelings of isolation, and promote a sense of community.
b. Improves Communication: Laughter breaks down barriers, eases tension, and encourages open communication among seniors. It can facilitate positive interactions and create a relaxed and comfortable social atmosphere.

4. Quality of Life:

a. Increases enjoyment: Laughter adds joy and happiness to seniors' lives, increasing their overall quality of life and making everyday activities more enjoyable.
b. Maintains a Positive Outlook: Laughter helps seniors maintain a positive perspective, enabling them to face life's challenges with resilience and optimism.
c. Promotes Well-rounded Wellness: Incorporating laughter into daily routines ensures a holistic approach to wellness, nurturing both physical and emotional well-being.

Incorporating laughter into fitness activities, social gatherings, and daily interactions can significantly contribute to the well-being of senior citizens. Laughter truly is a powerful tool for promoting wellness and enhancing the lives of seniors.

B. Introducing fun and lighthearted exercises

When it comes to creating a fun and lighthearted exercise book for senior citizens, there are several key factors to consider. Here are some ideas to get you started:

1. Warm-up activities:

Begin with gentle warm-up exercises that help seniors limber up and prepare their bodies for physical activity. This can include stretching, light cardio movements, and range-of-motion exercises.

2. Chair exercises:
Many seniors may have mobility issues or may prefer to exercise while seated. Include a variety of chair exercises that target different muscle groups, such as seated leg lifts, arm circles, and seated twists.

3. Balance and coordination exercises:
Focus on exercises that help improve balance and coordination, which are essential for preventing falls and maintaining independence. Examples may include standing on one leg, heel-to-toe walking, or using balance boards.

4. Flexibility exercises:
Include stretches and movements that promote flexibility and help seniors maintain or increase their range of motion. This can include gentle yoga poses, tai chi movements, or simple stretching routines.

5. Cognitive exercises:
Incorporate activities that stimulate the mind and promote cognitive health. This can include puzzles, memory games, trivia questions, or word exercises. Keeping the brain active is important for overall well-being.

6. Social activities:
Consider adding group activities or exercises that promote social interaction among seniors. This can include partner exercises, group walks, or group games that encourage conversation and camaraderie.

Remember to always prioritize safety and tailor the exercises to suit the abilities and needs of the seniors. It may be helpful to consult with a fitness professional or healthcare provider to ensure the exercises are appropriate. Good luck with your book, and I hope it brings joy and wellness to senior citizens!

C. <u>Enjoying the process and finding joy in every workout</u>

Making exercise enjoyable and finding joy in every workout is essential for senior citizens. Here are some tips to incorporate fun and lightheartedness into their exercise routines:

1. Music therapy:
Play upbeat and familiar music during workouts, as music has a positive impact on mood and motivation. Encourage seniors to move and groove to the rhythm, adding a fun element to their exercise routine.

2. Game-based exercises:
Integrate game-like activities into workouts to make them more engaging. This can include exercises like "Simon says," bean bag toss, balloon volleyball, or seated bowling. These games help seniors focus on the activity while having fun.

3. Group exercises:
Foster a sense of community and enjoyment by organizing group exercises. This can involve forming exercise clubs or workout classes specifically for seniors. Working out together in a supportive environment can make the process more enjoyable.

4. Outdoor activities:
Take advantage of outdoor spaces and nature by organizing exercises such as nature walks, gardening sessions, or group yoga classes in the park. Being surrounded by greenery and fresh air adds a refreshing and uplifting element to workouts.

5. Variety and creativity:
Keep workouts interesting by incorporating a variety of exercises and activities. This can include dance-based workouts, water aerobics, resistance band exercises, or even hula hooping. Trying something new and creative adds an element of excitement to the routine.

6. Celebrate milestones:

Encourage seniors to set goals and celebrate their achievements along the way. Recognize and acknowledge progress, whether it's increased strength, improved flexibility, or completing a challenging exercise. This boosts motivation and creates a positive and joyous atmosphere.

Remember, the goal is to make exercise enjoyable, safe, and beneficial for seniors. Always consider their individual needs and capabilities when designing the workouts. By adding fun and lightheartedness to their exercise routine, you can help seniors stay motivated, engaged, and ultimately enjoy the process of maintaining their health and well-being.

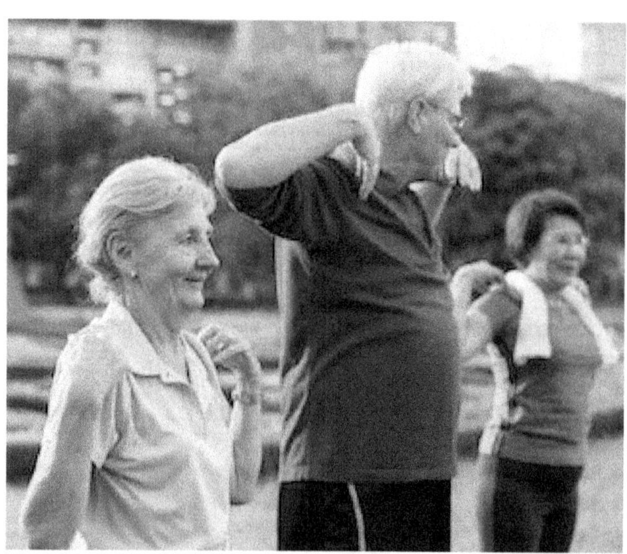

Chapter Six: How to Keep Senior Citizens Motivated and Consistent

Motivation and consistency are key factors in maintaining an active lifestyle for senior citizens. In this chapter, we will explore strategies and techniques to help seniors stay motivated and consistent with their exercise routines. By implementing these practices, you can support their long-term commitment to fitness, health, and overall well-being.

1. Set realistic and achievable goals:
Encourage seniors to set realistic and achievable goals that align with their abilities and interests. These goals should be specific, measurable, attainable, relevant, and time-bound (SMART). When goals are within reach, seniors are more likely to stay motivated and remain consistent in their efforts.

2. Tailor workouts to personal preferences:
Take into account seniors' personal preferences when designing their exercise routines. Whether it's dancing, swimming, walking, or practicing tai chi, tailoring workouts to their interests increases enjoyment and motivation. Allow for variety and flexibility in the types of exercises and activities offered.

3. Track progress:
Implement a system for tracking and recording progress. This can be as simple as keeping an exercise journal, using a fitness app, or utilizing a pedometer or activity tracker. Seeing improvements, however small, provides seniors with a sense of achievement and motivates them to continue their efforts.

4. Provide positive reinforcement:
Celebrate every milestone and achievement, no matter how small. Offer positive reinforcement and praise for their dedication and progress. This can be done through verbal encouragement, rewards, or recognition within the senior community. Positive feedback boosts motivation and encourages consistency.

5. Create a supportive environment:
Foster a supportive and encouraging environment that promotes social interaction and accountability. Encourage seniors to exercise with friends or join group classes where they can connect with like-minded individuals. Peer support and teamwork can help seniors stay motivated and consistent.

6. Adapt and modify routines:
As seniors age, their needs and abilities may change. It's important to adapt and modify exercise routines accordingly. Offering modifications and alternative exercises ensures that seniors can continue exercising safely and comfortably. Adjustments also prevent monotony, keeping workouts fresh and engaging.

7. Provide education and resources:
Educate seniors about the benefits of exercise and its impact on their health and well-being. Offer additional resources, such as informative articles, videos, or guest speakers, to enhance their understanding and motivation. The more seniors are informed, the more likely they are to stay motivated and consistent.

8. Regularly reassess and adjust:
Regularly reassess seniors' progress, goals, and preferences. Check for any changes in their physical abilities or interests. Modify their exercise routines accordingly to keep them engaged and motivated. Flexibility and adaptability are crucial in ensuring ongoing motivation and consistency.

By implementing these strategies and techniques, you can help senior citizens stay motivated and consistent with their exercise routines. Remember to be attentive to their individual needs, provide ongoing support, and keep the workouts enjoyable and varied. With your guidance and encouragement, seniors can maintain an active lifestyle and reap the numerous physical and mental benefits that regular exercise offers.

Note: It's important to consult with healthcare professionals or fitness experts when developing exercise routines for seniors to ensure their safety and suitability.

A. Setting realistic fitness goals

Setting realistic fitness goals for senior citizens is crucial to ensure their success, motivation, and overall well-being. Here are some guidelines to help you in this process:

1. Assess individual abilities:
Before setting any goals, assess the senior's current physical condition, medical history, and any limitations or considerations they may have. This will help you understand their abilities and set appropriate goals.

2. Focus on functional fitness:
Prioritize goals that enhance the senior's ability to perform everyday activities with ease and independence. Consider activities like walking, climbing stairs, maintaining balance, and improving flexibility. Functional fitness goals help seniors remain self-sufficient in their daily lives.

3. Start small and progress gradually:
Begin with attainable goals that are within the senior's reach. Starting with small milestones ensures success, builds confidence, and keeps motivation high. As they progress, gradually increase the intensity, duration, or complexity of the exercises to promote continuous improvement.

4. Use the SMART framework:
Set goals that follow the SMART framework - Specific, Measurable, Achievable, Relevant, and Time-bound. For example, instead of a vague goal like "improve strength," set a specific goal like "perform 10 bodyweight squats without assistance within 3 months." SMART goals provide clarity and help track progress effectively.

5. Consider short-term and long-term goals:
Encourage seniors to set both short-term and long-term goals. Short-term goals provide immediate motivation and a sense of accomplishment, while long-term goals offer a broader focus and help maintain consistency over

time. Ensure that each short-term goal aligns with the overarching long-term goal.

6. Personalize goals and preferences:
Involve seniors in the goal-setting process and consider their preferences. Ask them what they enjoy and what they would like to achieve. This personalization ensures that goals are meaningful to them, increasing their motivation to work towards them.

7. Celebrate milestones:
Recognize and celebrate every milestone achieved along the way. Acknowledge progress, whether it's an increase in strength, endurance, flexibility, or reaching a specific target. Celebrating milestones boosts confidence, motivates seniors, and encourages continued dedication.

8. Regularly reassess and adjust goals:
Periodically reassess the senior's progress and adjust goals accordingly. As their fitness level improves, continue setting new goals to challenge them. Be flexible and adaptive to their changing needs or preferences to keep them engaged and motivated.

Remember, the primary focus is on improving overall health, functional abilities, and quality of life for senior citizens. By setting realistic goals, you can help them achieve success, maintain motivation, and enjoy the benefits of an active and healthy lifestyle.

B. Creating a supportive environment

Creating a supportive environment for senior citizens is essential for their well-being and success in various aspects of life. Here are some ways to foster such an environment:

1. Communication and empathy:
Foster open and effective communication with seniors. Listen actively, show empathy, and validate their feelings and concerns. Create a safe space where they feel comfortable sharing their thoughts and needs.

2. Respect and dignity:
Treat seniors with respect and dignity, valuing their experiences and wisdom. Encourage others in the community to do the same. Create a culture that appreciates and celebrates the contributions of seniors.

3. Social connections:
Promote opportunities for social interactions among seniors. Organize social events, group activities, or clubs focused on shared interests. Encourage seniors to connect with one another, fostering a sense of belonging and companionship.

4. Volunteering and engagement:
Encourage seniors to participate in volunteer activities or community engagements. This can provide a sense of purpose, fulfillment, and social connection. Offer opportunities for them to contribute their skills, knowledge, and experiences to benefit others.

5. Health and wellness support:
Provide resources and support for seniors to maintain their physical and mental health. Offer fitness classes, health screenings, educational workshops, and access to healthcare professionals. Emphasize the importance of self-care and provide avenues for seniors to seek assistance when needed.

6. Lifelong learning:
Create an environment that encourages continuous learning and personal growth for seniors. Offer educational programs, workshops, book clubs, or lectures on a wide range of topics. Facilitate opportunities for seniors to expand their knowledge and engage in intellectual pursuits.

7. Safety and accessibility:
Ensure that the environment is safe, accessible, and accommodating to seniors' needs. This may include installing handrails, ramps, and proper lighting, or providing devices and technologies that aid mobility and

communication. Conduct regular assessments and updates to maintain a senior-friendly space.

8. Supportive staff and volunteers:
Train staff and volunteers to provide compassionate and respectful care for seniors. Ensure they understand the specific needs and challenges faced by seniors and have the skills to address them effectively. Encourage a team approach where everyone works together to support the well-being of seniors.

9. Regular feedback and improvement:
Seek feedback from seniors to understand their experiences and areas for improvement. Use this feedback to make necessary adjustments and enhancements to the environment, activities, and services provided. Continuously strive to create the best possible supportive environment.

By implementing these practices, you can create a supportive environment that values and nurtures senior citizens. This environment promotes their overall well-being, enhances their quality of life, and encourages them to live fulfilling and engaged lives.

Please note that while these suggestions can be helpful, it's important to tailor them to the specific needs and preferences of the seniors in your community. Every individual is unique and may require personalized support and adjustments.

C. Tracking progress and celebrating achievements

Tracking progress and celebrating achievements are essential for senior citizens to stay motivated and maintain a sense of accomplishment. Here are some ideas on how to do this effectively:

1. Establish measurable goals:
Set clear and measurable goals with seniors to track their progress. These goals can be related to fitness, mobility, cognitive abilities, or any other area of focus. For example, completing a certain number of steps in a day, increasing flexibility, or improving memory recall.

2. Record and track progress:
Use a tracking system to record the progress of seniors. This can be done through a simple journal or using technology like fitness apps or wearable devices. Track the frequency, duration, and intensity of exercises or activities, and record any improvements over time.

3. Provide visual representations:
Create charts, graphs, or visual representations of progress to help seniors visualize their achievements. Seeing their progress visually can be highly motivating and provide a sense of accomplishment. Share these visual representations regularly to reinforce their success.

4. Regular assessments and evaluations:
Conduct periodic assessments or evaluations to measure seniors' progress objectively. This can involve fitness tests, cognitive assessments, balance evaluations, or any other relevant measurement tool. Assessments provide concrete data and give seniors a clear understanding of their development.

5. Celebrate milestones and achievements:
Recognize and celebrate milestones and achievements along the way. Whether it's reaching a certain fitness goal, improving flexibility, or completing a cognitive challenge, acknowledge and congratulate seniors on their accomplishments. This can be done through verbal praise, certificates, or other forms of acknowledgment.

6. Share success stories:
Share success stories of seniors who have made significant progress or achieved their goals. This can inspire and motivate others within the senior community. Highlight their journey, challenges overcome, and the positive impact it had on their overall well-being.

7. Group celebrations:
Organize group celebrations or events to recognize the achievements of seniors collectively. This could be a monthly gathering, an annual awards ceremony, or a special event dedicated to celebrating their progress. Make it

a festive and enjoyable occasion that encourages social interaction and camaraderie.

8. Ongoing encouragement and support:
Provide continuous encouragement and support to seniors throughout their fitness journey. Offer positive feedback, reassurance, and motivation to keep them engaged and focused on their goals. Regularly check in with them to provide guidance, answer questions, and address any concerns.

Remember, each senior has unique capabilities and goals, so tailor the tracking and celebration process to their individual needs. By tracking progress and celebrating achievements, you empower seniors to recognize their progress, stay motivated, and continue striving for further improvements in their overall well-being.

Please note that while these suggestions can be helpful, it's important to consider any specific health concerns or limitations seniors may have. Consulting with healthcare professionals or fitness experts can provide valuable insights and personalized guidance.

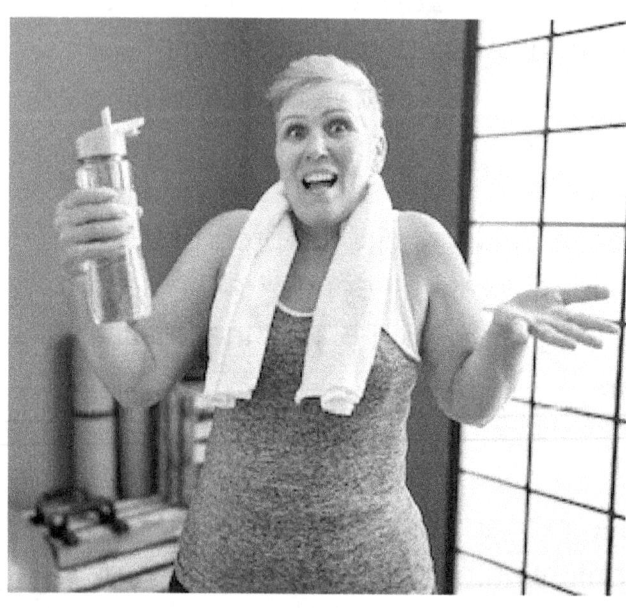

Chapter 7: Key Factors in Maintaining an Active Lifestyle

Motivation and consistency are key factors in maintaining an active lifestyle for senior citizens. In this chapter, we will explore strategies and techniques to help seniors stay motivated and consistent with their exercise routines. By implementing these practices, you can support their long-term commitment to fitness, health, and overall well-being.

1. Set realistic and achievable goals:
Encourage seniors to set realistic and achievable goals that align with their abilities and interests. These goals should be specific, measurable, attainable, relevant, and time-bound (SMART). When goals are within reach, seniors are more likely to stay motivated and remain consistent in their efforts.

2. Tailor workouts to personal preferences:
Take into account seniors' personal preferences when designing their exercise routines. Whether it's dancing, swimming, walking, or practicing tai chi, tailoring workouts to their interests increases enjoyment and motivation. Allow for variety and flexibility in the types of exercises and activities offered.

3. Track progress:
Implement a system for tracking and recording progress. This can be as simple as keeping an exercise journal, using a fitness app, or utilizing a pedometer or activity tracker. Seeing improvements, however small, provides seniors with a sense of achievement and motivates them to continue their efforts.

4. Provide positive reinforcement:
Celebrate every milestone and achievement, no matter how small. Offer positive reinforcement and praise for their dedication and progress. This can be done through verbal encouragement, rewards, or recognition within the senior community. Positive feedback boosts motivation and encourages consistency.

5. Create a supportive environment:

Foster a supportive and encouraging environment that promotes social interaction and accountability. Encourage seniors to exercise with friends or join group classes where they can connect with like-minded individuals. Peer support and teamwork can help seniors stay motivated and consistent.

6. Adapt and modify routines:
As seniors age, their needs and abilities may change. It's important to adapt and modify exercise routines accordingly. Offering modifications and alternative exercises ensures that seniors can continue exercising safely and comfortably. Adjustments also prevent monotony, keeping workouts fresh and engaging.

7. Provide education and resources:
Educate seniors about the benefits of exercise and its impact on their health and well-being. Offer additional resources, such as informative articles, videos, or guest speakers, to enhance their understanding and motivation. The more seniors are informed, the more likely they are to stay motivated and consistent.

8. Regularly reassess and adjust:
Regularly reassess seniors' progress, goals, and preferences. Check for any changes in their physical abilities or interests. Modify their exercise routines accordingly to keep them engaged and motivated. Flexibility and adaptability are crucial in ensuring ongoing motivation and consistency.

By implementing these strategies and techniques, you can help senior citizens stay motivated and consistent with their exercise routines. Remember to be attentive to their individual needs, provide ongoing support, and keep the workouts enjoyable and varied. With your guidance and encouragement, seniors can maintain an active lifestyle and reap the numerous physical and mental benefits that regular exercise offers.

Note: It's important to consult with healthcare professionals or fitness experts when developing exercise routines for seniors to ensure their safety and suitability.

A. Setting realistic fitness goals

Setting realistic fitness goals for senior citizens is crucial to ensure their success, motivation, and overall well-being. Here are some guidelines to help you in this process:

1. Assess individual abilities:
Before setting any goals, assess the senior's current physical condition, medical history, and any limitations or considerations they may have. This will help you understand their abilities and set appropriate goals.

2. Focus on functional fitness:
Prioritize goals that enhance the senior's ability to perform everyday activities with ease and independence. Consider activities like walking, climbing stairs, maintaining balance, and improving flexibility. Functional fitness goals help seniors remain self-sufficient in their daily lives.

3. Start small and progress gradually:
Begin with attainable goals that are within the senior's reach. Starting with small milestones ensures success, builds confidence, and keeps motivation high. As they progress, gradually increase the intensity, duration, or complexity of the exercises to promote continuous improvement.

4. Use the SMART framework:
Set goals that follow the SMART framework - Specific, Measurable, Achievable, Relevant, and Time-bound. For example, instead of a vague goal like "improve strength," set a specific goal like "perform 10 bodyweight squats without assistance within 3 months." SMART goals provide clarity and help track progress effectively.

5. Consider short-term and long-term goals:
Encourage seniors to set both short-term and long-term goals. Short-term goals provide immediate motivation and a sense of accomplishment, while long-term goals offer a broader focus and help maintain consistency over time. Ensure that each short-term goal aligns with the overarching long-term goal.

6. Personalize goals and preferences:
Involve seniors in the goal-setting process and consider their preferences. Ask them what they enjoy and what they would like to achieve. This personalization ensures that goals are meaningful to them, increasing their motivation to work towards them.

7. Celebrate milestones:
Recognize and celebrate every milestone achieved along the way. Acknowledge progress, whether it's an increase in strength, endurance, flexibility, or reaching a specific target. Celebrating milestones boosts confidence, motivates seniors, and encourages continued dedication.

8. Regularly reassess and adjust goals:
Periodically reassess the senior's progress and adjust goals accordingly. As their fitness level improves, continue setting new goals to challenge them. Be flexible and adaptive to their changing needs or preferences to keep them engaged and motivated.

Remember, the primary focus is on improving overall health, functional abilities, and quality of life for senior citizens. By setting realistic goals, you can help them achieve success, maintain motivation, and enjoy the benefits of an active and healthy lifestyle.

B. <u>Creating a supportive environment</u>

Creating a supportive environment for senior citizens is essential for their well-being and success in various aspects of life. Here are some ways to foster such an environment:

1. Communication and empathy:
Foster open and effective communication with seniors. Listen actively, show empathy, and validate their feelings and concerns. Create a safe space where they feel comfortable sharing their thoughts and needs.

2. Respect and dignity:

Treat seniors with respect and dignity, valuing their experiences and wisdom.
Encourage others in the community to do the same. Create a culture that
appreciates and celebrates the contributions of seniors.

3. Social connections:
Promote opportunities for social interactions among seniors. Organize social
events, group activities, or clubs focused on shared interests. Encourage
seniors to connect with one another, fostering a sense of belonging and
companionship.

4. Volunteering and engagement:
Encourage seniors to participate in volunteer activities or community
engagements. This can provide a sense of purpose, fulfillment, and social
connection. Offer opportunities for them to contribute their skills, knowledge,
and experiences to benefit others.

5. Health and wellness support:
Provide resources and support for seniors to maintain their physical and
mental health. Offer fitness classes, health screenings, educational
workshops, and access to healthcare professionals. Emphasize the
importance of self-care and provide avenues for seniors to seek assistance
when needed.

6. Lifelong learning:
Create an environment that encourages continuous learning and personal
growth for seniors. Offer educational programs, workshops, book clubs, or
lectures on a wide range of topics. Facilitate opportunities for seniors to
expand their knowledge and engage in intellectual pursuits.

7. Safety and accessibility:
Ensure that the environment is safe, accessible, and accommodating to
seniors' needs. This may include installing handrails, ramps, and proper
lighting, or providing devices and technologies that aid mobility and
communication. Conduct regular assessments and updates to maintain a
senior-friendly space.

8. Supportive staff and volunteers:
Train staff and volunteers to provide compassionate and respectful care for seniors. Ensure they understand the specific needs and challenges faced by seniors and have the skills to address them effectively. Encourage a team approach where everyone works together to support the well-being of seniors.

9. Regular feedback and improvement:
Seek feedback from seniors to understand their experiences and areas for improvement. Use this feedback to make necessary adjustments and enhancements to the environment, activities, and services provided. Continuously strive to create the best possible supportive environment.

By implementing these practices, you can create a supportive environment that values and nurtures senior citizens. This environment promotes their overall well-being, enhances their quality of life, and encourages them to live fulfilling and engaged lives.

Please note that while these suggestions can be helpful, it's important to tailor them to the specific needs and preferences of the seniors in your community. Every individual is unique and may require personalized support and adjustments.

C. <u>Tracking progress and celebrating achievements</u>

Tracking progress and celebrating achievements is essential for senior citizens to stay motivated and maintain a sense of accomplishment. Here are some ideas on how to do this effectively:

1. Establish measurable goals:
Set clear and measurable goals with seniors to track their progress. These goals can be related to fitness, mobility, cognitive abilities, or any other area of focus. For example, completing a certain number of steps in a day, increasing flexibility, or improving memory recall.

2. Record and track progress:

Use a tracking system to record the progress of seniors. This can be done through a simple journal or using technology like fitness apps or wearable devices. Track the frequency, duration, and intensity of exercises or activities, and record any improvements over time.

3. Provide visual representations:
Create charts, graphs, or visual representations of progress to help seniors visualize their achievements. Seeing their progress visually can be highly motivating and provide a sense of accomplishment. Share these visual representations regularly to reinforce their success.

4. Regular assessments and evaluations:
Conduct periodic assessments or evaluations to measure seniors' progress objectively. This can involve fitness tests, cognitive assessments, balance evaluations, or any other relevant measurement tool. Assessments provide concrete data and give seniors a clear understanding of their development.

5. Celebrate milestones and achievements:
Recognize and celebrate milestones and achievements along the way. Whether it's reaching a certain fitness goal, improving flexibility, or completing a cognitive challenge, acknowledge and congratulate seniors on their accomplishments. This can be done through verbal praise, certificates, or other forms of acknowledgment.

6. Share success stories:
Share success stories of seniors who have made significant progress or achieved their goals. This can inspire and motivate others within the senior community. Highlight their journey, challenges overcome, and the positive impact it had on their overall well-being.

7. Group celebrations:
Organize group celebrations or events to recognize the achievements of seniors collectively. This could be a monthly gathering, an annual awards ceremony, or a special event dedicated to celebrating their progress. Make it a festive and enjoyable occasion that encourages social interaction and camaraderie.

8. Ongoing encouragement and support:
Provide continuous encouragement and support to seniors throughout their fitness journey. Offer positive feedback, reassurance, and motivation to keep them engaged and focused on their goals. Regularly check in with them to provide guidance, answer questions, and address any concerns.

Remember, each senior has unique capabilities and goals, so tailor the tracking and celebration process to their individual needs. By tracking progress and celebrating achievements, you empower seniors to recognize their progress, stay motivated, and continue striving for further improvements in their overall well-being.

Please note that while these suggestions can be helpful, it's important to consider any specific health concerns or limitations seniors may have. Consulting with healthcare professionals or fitness experts can provide valuable insights and personalized guidance.

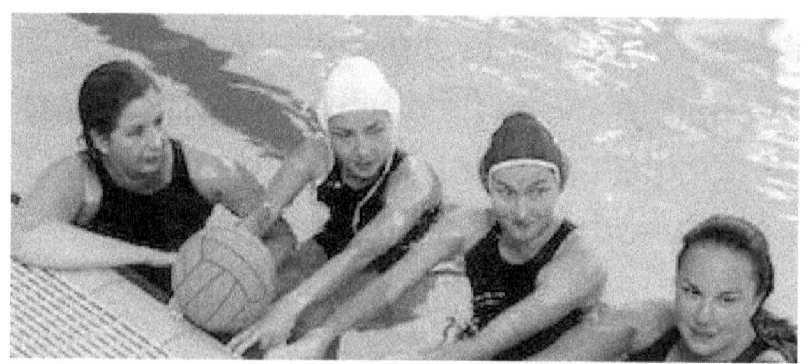

<u>Chapter 8: Additional Tips and Resources</u>

In Chapter 7, we discussed various exercises that are beneficial for senior citizens. In this chapter, we will provide additional tips and resources to help seniors make the most out of their exercise routines. These tips will focus on safety, motivation, and accessing helpful resources.

1. Safety First:
Exercise is important, but it's equally crucial to prioritize safety, especially for senior citizens. Here are a few safety tips to keep in mind:

a. Consult with a healthcare professional:
Before starting any exercise program, it is advisable to consult with a healthcare professional, particularly if you have any pre-existing medical conditions or concerns.

b. Warm-up and cool-down:
Begin each exercise session with a gentle warm-up to prepare your body for activity. Also, remember to cool down afterward to gradually lower your heart rate and stretch your muscles.

c. Stay hydrated:
Drink plenty of water before, during, and after exercising to prevent dehydration.

d. Use proper equipment and attire:
Wear comfortable clothing and supportive shoes that provide stability and prevent falls. If necessary, use any recommended assistive devices, such as walking aids or braces.

e. Listen to your body:
Pay attention to any pain or discomfort during exercise. If something doesn't feel right, modify, or stop the activity and consult your healthcare professional if needed.

2. <u>Motivation and Enjoyment:</u>

Staying motivated and enjoying your exercise routine can make a significant difference. Here are some tips to keep you motivated:

a. Set realistic goals:
Establish achievable short-term and long-term exercise goals that align with your capabilities. Celebrate your progress along the way.

b. Find an exercise buddy:
Exercising with a friend or family member can provide motivation, accountability, and companionship.

c. Try different activities:
Variety can help prevent boredom and keep you engaged. Explore different forms of exercise, such as walking, swimming, tai chi, or yoga, to discover what you enjoy the most.

d. Join a senior-specific fitness program:
Look for fitness classes or programs designed specifically for senior citizens. They often provide a supportive environment and cater to the needs of older adults.

e. Track your progress:
Keep a record of your exercise routine, including activities, duration, and any improvements or milestones achieved. It can help motivate you and provide a sense of accomplishment.

3. Accessing Resources:
Several resources are available to help senior citizens with their exercise journey. Here are a few worth exploring:

a. Local community centers or senior centers:
Check if your local community or senior center offers exercise classes or programs tailored for seniors. They may provide affordable options and a chance to socialize with like-minded individuals.

b. Online exercise videos:

The internet offers a wealth of exercise videos specifically designed for seniors. Websites like YouTube have a wide range of low-impact exercise routines that can be performed at home.

c. Senior fitness apps:
Consider downloading fitness apps designed for older adults. These apps offer guided exercises, progress tracking, and reminders to help you stay on track.

d. Senior-specific fitness organizations:
Explore organizations like Silver Sneakers, Silver&Fit, or the National Institute on Aging for resources and information on senior fitness.

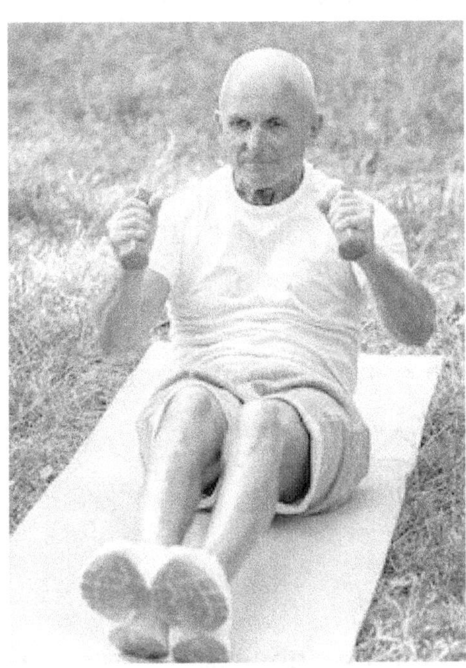

By prioritizing safety, finding motivation, and accessing relevant resources, senior citizens can enhance their exercise experience and reap the numerous benefits it provides. Remember to consult with a healthcare professional, listen to your body, and enjoy the process. Age is just a number, and regular exercise can contribute to improved overall health and well-being.

A. Healthy lifestyle recommendations for seniors

Maintaining a healthy lifestyle is crucial for seniors to promote overall well-being. Here are some important recommendations:

1. Balanced Diet:
- Consume a variety of nutrient-dense foods, including fruits, vegetables, whole grains, lean proteins, and low-fat dairy products.
- Limit the intake of processed foods, sugary snacks, and beverages with added sugars.
- Stay hydrated by drinking plenty of water throughout the day.

2. Regular Exercise:
- Engage in regular physical activity, as recommended by your healthcare professional. Aim for a combination of aerobic exercises, strength training, and balance exercises.
- Find activities that you enjoy and consider incorporating them into your routine, such as walking, swimming, dancing, or tai chi.
- Start slowly and gradually increase the intensity and duration of your exercises.

3. Adequate Sleep:
- Aim for 7-8 hours of quality sleep each night. Maintain a consistent sleep schedule and create a comfortable sleeping environment.
- Avoid caffeine and electronic devices close to bedtime, as they can interfere with sleep.

4. Social Connections:
- Stay socially active and maintain regular interactions with family, friends, and community members.
- Join clubs, volunteer, or participate in activities that interest you to foster social connections and combat feelings of loneliness.

5. Mental Stimulation:
- Engage in activities that stimulate your mind, such as reading, puzzles, crosswords, learning new skills, or pursuing hobbies.
- Stay mentally active by engaging in social conversations, taking educational courses, or using brain-training apps.

6. Regular Health Check-ups:
- Schedule regular check-ups with your healthcare provider to monitor your overall health, manage any existing medical conditions, and update vaccinations.
- Follow prescribed medication regimens and communicate any concerns or changes in your health to your healthcare professional.

7. Stress Management:
- Practice stress-reducing techniques, such as deep breathing exercises, meditation, yoga, or engaging in activities that help you relax and unwind.
- Seek emotional support from loved ones or consider joining support groups to cope with any stress or anxiety.

8. Fall Prevention:
- Create a safe living environment by removing potential hazards, using handrails, installing grab bars in bathrooms, and ensuring proper lighting.
- Wear appropriate footwear with good traction, consider mobility aids if needed, and participate in balance exercises to reduce the risk of falls.

Remember, it's essential to consult with your healthcare professional before making any significant lifestyle changes or starting a new exercise program. They can provide personalized guidance based on your specific health needs and limitations.

B. <u>Exploring technology and fitness apps for seniors</u>

Exploring technology and fitness apps can be a great way for seniors to enhance their exercise routines and overall health. Here are some popular fitness apps specifically designed for seniors:

1. SilverSneakers GO:
Available for iPhone and Android, this app offers guided exercise routines suitable for seniors. It provides instructional videos for various workout types, including cardio, strength, and flexibility exercises.

2. MyFitnessPal:
This widely used app helps users track their nutrition and exercise. It allows seniors to set health goals, monitor calorie intake, and track exercise progress. The app is available for both iPhone and Android.

3. Aaptiv:
Aaptiv offers audio-based workout programs for users of all fitness levels. With a wide range of options, including guided walks, running, cycling, and strength training, seniors can find personalized workout routines to fit their needs. The app is available for iPhone and Android.

4. Fitbod:
Fitbod is a strength training app that provides customized workout plans based on individual goals, preferences, and available equipment. The app takes into account factors like age and fitness level to create safe and effective workout routines. It is available for iPhone and Android.

5. Yoga for Seniors:
This app focuses on gentle yoga exercises suitable for seniors. It offers various yoga routines, designed to improve flexibility, balance, and strength. Yoga for Seniors is available for both iPhone and Android.

6. BrainHQ:
Developed by Posit Science, BrainHQ offers a wide range of brain-training exercises to enhance cognitive function and mental sharpness. The app provides personalized workouts designed to improve memory, attention, and overall brain health. It is available for both iPhone and Android.

Note that the availability and features of apps may change over time, so it's always a good idea to check the respective app stores or websites for the latest information.

Additionally, seniors may benefit from other useful technologies such as fitness trackers and smartwatches, which can monitor heart rate, sleep patterns, and activity levels. These devices often come with corresponding apps that provide valuable insights into fitness progress.

Remember, it's important to choose apps that align with your specific needs, preferences, and fitness level. Consult with your healthcare professional or a trusted source if you need assistance in selecting the most suitable apps and technologies for your exercise routine.

C. Seeking professional assistance and guidance

Seeking professional assistance and guidance is highly recommended for senior citizens when it comes to exercising. Here are some professionals who can provide valuable support:

1. Primary Care Physician:
Consult with your primary care physician or a geriatrician before starting any exercise program, especially if you have pre-existing medical conditions or concerns. They can assess your overall health and provide guidance on exercise options suitable for your specific needs.

2. Physical Therapist:
 A physical therapist can assess your physical abilities, mobility, and any specific limitations or concerns. They can design personalized exercise programs, teach you proper techniques, and provide guidance on preventing injuries.

3. Certified Personal Trainer:
Working with a certified personal trainer with experience in senior fitness can provide tailored exercise programs to meet your needs and goals. They can

ensure that exercises are performed correctly and safely, and gradually progress your routines as you improve.

4. Exercise Physiologist:
An exercise physiologist specializes in developing exercise programs based on your needs and health conditions. They can help you address specific health concerns, such as cardiovascular issues, diabetes, or arthritis, and create exercise plans that work within those parameters.

5. Senior Fitness Specialist:
A senior fitness specialist is trained specifically to work with older adults and understands the unique needs and considerations of seniors. They can provide specialized guidance and modifications for exercises, keeping in mind any age-related physical changes and limitations.

6. Group Exercise Instructors:
Joining group exercise classes led by qualified instructors can offer a supportive environment and social interaction. Look for classes designed specifically for seniors, such as water aerobics, yoga, or tai chi, that are led by instructors experienced in working with older adults.

Remember, these professionals can offer personalized guidance based on your specific health conditions and needs. Always communicate openly about any concerns or limitations you may have and be sure to follow their recommendations for safe and effective exercise routines.

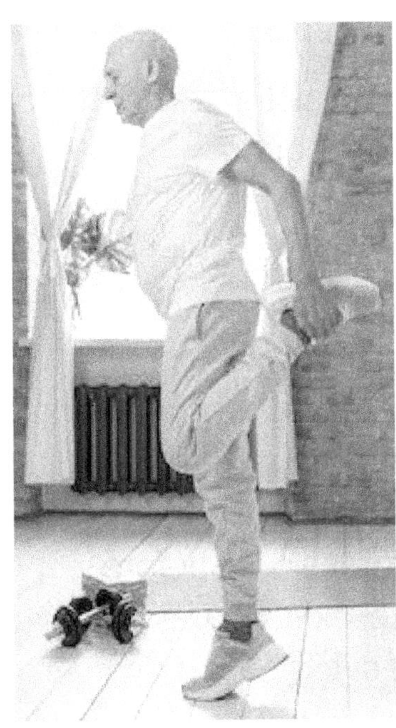

In this book, we have explored the importance of exercise for senior citizens and provided valuable information to help seniors incorporate exercise into their lives. We discussed various types of exercises suitable for seniors, including aerobic activities, strength training, balance exercises, and flexibility exercises.

Throughout the chapters, we emphasized the numerous benefits of exercise for seniors, including improved cardiovascular health, increased strength and mobility, enhanced balance and coordination, better mental health, and a reduced risk of chronic diseases and falls. We also offered tips and guidance on how to get started with an exercise routine, adapt exercises to individual needs, and overcome common barriers to exercise.

Safety was a significant focus, as we highlighted the importance of consulting with healthcare professionals, warming up and cooling down properly, using appropriate equipment and attire, and listening to one's body during exercise. We also stressed the significance of motivation and enjoyment in sustaining an exercise routine and suggested setting realistic goals, finding exercise buddies, trying different activities, tracking progress, and accessing senior-specific fitness programs and resources.

Additionally, we touched upon the role of technology in supporting senior fitness, recommending fitness apps and devices that can assist in tracking progress, providing guided workouts, and promoting brain health.

In conclusion, exercise is vital for promoting physical and mental well-being, and senior citizens can experience numerous benefits by incorporating regular exercise into their lives. By following the guidelines, seeking professional guidance when needed, prioritizing safety, and enjoying the process, seniors can embark on a journey towards healthier and more active lifestyles.

Remember, it's important to consult with a healthcare professional before starting any exercise program, particularly if you have pre-existing medical conditions or concerns. They can provide personalized advice based on your health status.

As always, fostering a healthy and active lifestyle is a continuous journey. We hope this book has provided you with valuable insights and tools to embrace exercise and its benefits fully. Start small, stay committed, and enjoy the rewards that exercise can bring.

A. <u>Recap of the benefits of a regular 5-minute fitness routine for seniors</u>

1. Improved cardiovascular health:
Engaging in brief aerobic exercises, such as brisk walking or marching in place, can help elevate heart rate and strengthen the cardiovascular system. This contributes to improved heart health and better circulation.

2. Increased mobility and flexibility:
Performing gentle stretches and mobility exercises for various muscle groups can enhance flexibility and range of motion. This can help seniors maintain functional independence and reduce the risk of joint stiffness and muscle imbalances.

3. Enhanced muscle strength:
Incorporating resistance exercises, like bodyweight squats or light dumbbell exercises, into a 5-minute routine can improve muscle strength and tone.

Strong muscles support better balance, stability, and overall functional abilities.

4. Boosted mood and mental well-being:
Even a short exercise session can stimulate the release of endorphins, which are natural mood enhancers. Regular physical activity can also reduce symptoms of depression and anxiety, improve cognitive function, and promote better sleep.

5. Reduced risk of chronic conditions:
Engaging in regular physical activity, even for just 5 minutes a day, can help lower the risk of chronic conditions such as heart disease, diabetes, and certain types of cancer. It can also aid in weight management and promote healthy aging.

6. Improved balance and fall prevention:
Incorporating balance exercises, such as standing on one leg or practicing heel-to-toe walking, can enhance balance and stability. This is essential for preventing falls, which can be particularly harmful for seniors.

Remember, while a 5-minute routine can offer benefits, it is important to gradually increase the duration and intensity of exercise as tolerated. Always consult with a healthcare professional before starting any exercise program, especially if you have pre-existing medical conditions or concerns.

B. <u>Encouragement to take the first step towards a healthier and happier life</u>

As a senior citizen, taking the first step towards a healthier and happier life can bring about incredible positive changes. It's never too late to prioritize your well-being and embrace a new chapter filled with vitality and joy.

1. Embrace the Power of Now:
Remember that every moment is an opportunity to make a positive change. Don't let age be a barrier; instead, let it fuel your determination to make the most out of every day.

2. Start Small, Dream Big:
Begin by setting achievable goals that align with your aspirations. Whether it's going for a daily walk, joining a fitness class, or exploring a new hobby, taking small steps in the right direction will gradually build momentum towards a healthier lifestyle.

3. Cultivate a Supportive Network:
Surround yourself with people who uplift and inspire you. Joining community groups or senior centers can provide a valuable support system and foster meaningful connections that enable you to share your journey with like-minded individuals.

4. Prioritize Self-Care:
Remember that taking care of yourself is not selfish but rather a powerful act of self-love. Incorporate self-care activities into your routine, such as meditation, mindfulness exercises, hobbies, or leisurely walks in nature. Nourishing your mind, body, and soul will strengthen your overall well-being.

5. Embrace New Opportunities:
Stay open to trying new things and exploring uncharted territories. Learning a new skill, traveling to new destinations, or volunteering for a cause you believe in can bring immense fulfillment and a renewed sense of purpose.

6. Celebrate Milestones:
Acknowledge and celebrate the milestones you achieve along the way. Each small success is worth recognizing and will provide the motivation to keep pushing forward.

Remember, it's never too late to embark on a journey towards a healthier and happier life. With determination, support, and self-care, you can create a fulfilling and vibrant chapter filled with new adventures, personal growth, and joy.

THE END
(or maybe just the beginning for you?!)

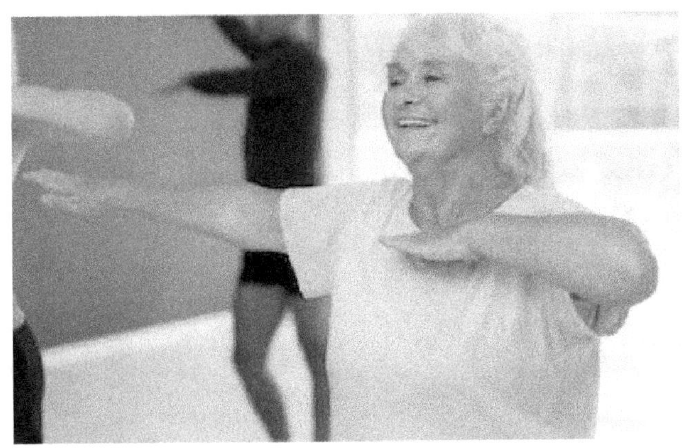

If you found this book helpful, please leave a positive review on Amazon.